I0093094

SLEEP MASTERY

The Complete Guide to Overcoming Insomnia, Increasing Energy, and Maximizing Daily Focus

KILEY MANNING

© **Copyright Kiley Manning 2025 - All rights reserved.**
This book is protected under copyright law and intended for personal use only. Any reproduction, distribution, or modification of its content without prior written consent from the author or publisher is prohibited.

ISBN: 978-1-923422-01-8

Disclaimer:
The information in this book is for educational and entertainment purposes and is not intended as legal, financial, medical, or professional advice. While efforts have been made to ensure accuracy as of 2025, no guarantees are made regarding the content's completeness or applicability.

Readers should consult licensed professionals before applying any techniques or strategies discussed. The author and publisher are not responsible for any outcomes, losses, or consequences resulting from the use of this book's information.

Table of Contents

Introduction

Sleep is a cornerstone of health and well-being, acting as a nightly reset that allows our minds and bodies to function properly. Yet, for many, achieving quality rest can feel elusive. Stress, lifestyle habits, and environmental factors often stand in the way, but with the right knowledge and strategies, you can overcome these obstacles and get the sleep your body craves.

Far from being a passive state, sleep is a dynamic process where vital functions take place. During this time, your body repairs tissues, balances hormones, and processes memories, laying the foundation for physical and mental health. Consistently missing out on sleep doesn't just leave you tired—it puts your health at risk, increasing the likelihood of anxiety, depression, impaired cognitive function, heart disease, and metabolic issues.

This book is your comprehensive guide to understanding and optimizing your sleep patterns. From exploring the principles of good sleep hygiene to uncovering practical techniques for deeper, more restorative rest, you'll gain actionable insights to transform your nights. We'll discuss the role of diet and lifestyle in promoting better sleep, delve into common disorders like insomnia and sleep apnea, and offer guidance on when to seek professional help.

Getting good sleep isn't a luxury—it's a necessity. By prioritizing rest, you can improve your energy, emotional well-being, productivity, and overall quality of life. This book doesn't just explain the "what" and "why" of sleep but also provides the "how"—realistic, research-backed strategies that fit into any schedule or lifestyle.

By the time you finish, you'll feel equipped with the tools to reclaim your nights, wake up refreshed, and approach each day ready to thrive. Your journey to better sleep starts here, and I'm excited to help guide you along the way.

- Kiley Manning

Many things—such as loving, going to sleep,
or behaving unaffectedly—are done worst
when we try hardest to do them.

- C.S. Lewis

Chapter 1

The Science of Sleep

Sleep, from an outside perspective, might seem straightforward: we close our eyes, drift off, and eventually wake up...

...But for those of us struggling with sleep, it often feels anything but simple. The truth is, sleep is a complex process, and many factors influence whether we experience restful or restless nights.

Understanding what happens in our brain and body during these hours can give us insight into the barriers we face and help us make gentle adjustments to our habits and environment, creating a better opportunity for restful sleep.

So, for this chapter, let's begin by going over the basics of sleep...

1.1 Understanding Sleep Mechanics

The moment you tuck yourself into bed and turn the lights off, your body, right before it shuts down for the day, will begin initiating a complex cycle that is as critical as any part of your waking life—each representing a phase of sleep and each with its own purpose.

Light Sleep

The first stage you'll enter is what's known as light sleep, also referred to as non-REM stage one. This sleep phase is typically the transition between wakefulness and sleep, making it easier to be awakened compared to later stages.

During light sleep, your heart rate begins to slow, and your breathing becomes more even and rhythmic. Your muscles may experience sudden twitches or contractions, a phenomenon called hypnic jerks, which are common as your body relaxes.

Gradually, your brain waves start to shift from an alert, active state to slower, more relaxed patterns. This is also when your thoughts begin to drift, and your mind lets go of the day's stressors, preparing you to move deeper into the restorative stages of sleep.

It should be noted that this stage of sleep is easy to wake from and may cause sleeplessness if you don't wind down properly and prepare your body for a long night of sleep.

Deep Sleep: Non-REM Stage 3

By the time you enter the first deep sleep stage, also known as non-REM stage three, your body begins a crucial repair and recovery process.

During this stage, your body goes into full 'repair mode,' addressing the wear and tear that your brain and body have experienced throughout the day. Growth hormones are released in greater quantities, which are essential for repairing damaged muscles and tissues, promoting overall physical recovery, and supporting growth in children and adolescents.

Additionally, this stage plays a vital role in boosting immune functions, as your body produces more immune cells to fight infections and improve resistance to illness.

The deep sleep stage is when your brain also clears out metabolic waste products, allowing it to recover and recharge for optimal function the next day. This period of deep, slow-wave sleep is fundamental to maintaining your physical health and mental well-being, ensuring your body is well-equipped to handle the challenges of the following day.

The deep sleep stage is also relatively harder to wake up once you've reached it—not waking from this stage will mean your body is deeply immersed in the restorative process.

Rapid Eye Movement Sleep

The sleep cycle progresses into Rapid Eye Movement (REM) sleep, a truly fascinating stage where the magic of dreaming comes alive. During this phase, your brain activity increases significantly, becoming almost as lively as when you're awake, which is why REM sleep is sometimes called 'paradoxical sleep.' This heightened activity allows your mind to engage in vivid dreams, where the thoughts and experiences of your day are creatively woven into story-like sequences.

But REM sleep isn't just about dreams—it's an essential period for cognitive and emotional processing. Your brain is hard at work "organizing" the mental files of your day, sorting through all the experiences, emotions, and information you've gathered. This is when the mind decides what to keep and store as long-term memories and what to discard as unnecessary details.

Essentially, REM sleep plays a critical role in memory consolidation, learning, and emotional regulation, helping you make sense of your world and retain important information. During this stage, your body also experiences temporary muscle paralysis, which prevents you from physically acting out your dreams, keeping you safe as your imagination takes flight. In this way, REM sleep is crucial for maintaining mental clarity, emotional balance, and overall cognitive health.

Complete Sleep Cycle

As your sleep continues, your body moves through multiple cycles, transitioning back and forth between deep sleep and REM sleep in a rhythmic pattern throughout the night. During each sleep cycle, you experience a delicate balance of different stages—ranging from light sleep to restorative deep sleep and the more active REM sleep.

Deep sleep is an important component of physical recovery and repair, where your body works on regenerating cells, strengthening your immune system, and solidifying any growth processes. It's during these cycles that your muscles fully relax, your heart rate and breathing are at their lowest, and your body gets the rest it needs to restore itself physically.

After each deep sleep phase, you gradually enter REM sleep, which allows your brain to process the day's experiences, emotions, and memories. This alternation between deep sleep and REM sleep helps you benefit from both physical and mental restoration needed for optimal well-being. Throughout the night, the time you spend in REM sleep lengthens while deep sleep shortens, which is why REM becomes more dominant in the early morning hours.

Finally, as you reach the later part of your sleep cycle, your body enters the late deep sleep stage. By this point, your mind has largely completed its processing, and your body has had a chance to carry out its restorative functions. The late deep sleep phase ensures that your energy is replenished, leaving you ready to wake up refreshed and ready to face a new day.

This continuous cycle of transitioning between deep sleep and REM sleep is fundamental for maintaining both mental and physical health, ensuring that you achieve the quality rest your body and mind need.

1.2 Acute vs. Chronic Insomnia

Insomnia is not just a blanket term for sleep troubles—it's a complex condition that has affected millions, making the simple act of falling asleep feel like an impossible task for most. At its core, insomnia involves difficulty in falling asleep, staying asleep, or waking up either at night or too early in the morning and being unable to go back to sleep. Some folks might even find themselves tossing and turning a few nights a month, while others might wrestle with sleep almost every single night.

And while it's often seen as a nighttime issue, its effects ripple into daylight hours, impacting energy levels, mood, and overall quality of life.

There are different types of insomnia, each with its nuances and challenges, and knowing them better can help you accurately pinpoint what's messing with your sleep pattern, namely, acute and chronic insomnia.

Acute Insomnia

Acute insomnia is a short-term visitor—a temporary disruption in your sleep patterns that often catches you off guard. It's the kind of sleeplessness that typically shows up during times of heightened stress or following a significant life event. Imagine the restless nights before an important job interview, the anxiety that accompanies a big move to a new city, or the nervous anticipation before an upcoming test. These moments of stress and uncertainty can make it difficult for your mind to settle, keeping you awake as you replay scenarios or imagine what's to come.

Acute insomnia isn't limited to moments of stress alone; it can also arise from other temporary changes in your environment or routine. For instance, jet lag from travel, an unexpected illness, or even a change in your work schedule can all contribute to short-term difficulties falling or staying asleep. The body may struggle to adapt to these sudden changes, and as a result, your sleep may be affected.

Fortunately, acute insomnia usually resolves once the stressor fades or your routine returns to normal. It often lasts just a few days to a few weeks, allowing you to eventually return to a regular sleep pattern once the cause of the disruption has passed. Unlike chronic insomnia, acute insomnia doesn't tend to linger—it's a fleeting reaction to specific circumstances, and once you address the cause, your sleep is likely to improve.

Chronic Insomnia

Chronic insomnia—the long-term visitor—is on the other end of the spectrum. Unlike acute insomnia, which passes with changing circumstances, chronic insomnia can linger for months or, in worst-case scenarios, even years. It's defined as lasting at least three months and occurring at least three nights a week, making it a persistent and exhausting challenge for those who suffer from it. The effects of chronic insomnia are far-reaching and go well beyond just feeling tired during the day; its long-lasting presence can deeply impact both physical and mental health, leading to a cascade of stress, emotional turmoil, and even more serious health conditions.

Chronic insomnia often becomes a vicious cycle, where the more you struggle with sleep, the more anxiety and frustration you feel around bedtime. This sleep anxiety can perpetuate sleeplessness, leading to increased emotional distress and an ongoing sense of helplessness. As nights of restless tossing and turning become the norm, the body and mind enter a state of heightened alertness, making it even harder to fall asleep naturally. Over time, this pattern can significantly affect one's mood, leading to irritability, anxiety, or even depression.

The long-term effects of chronic insomnia don't stop there. Sleep not only plays an important role in maintaining our overall health, but also heavily supports the immune system in regulating metabolism and allowing the brain to process information. When sleep is continually disrupted, the body misses out on these vital restorative processes. Chronic insomnia can, therefore, contribute to health issues like high blood pressure, weakened immunity, weight gain, and an increased risk of developing conditions such as diabetes or cardiovascular disease.

The causes of chronic insomnia are often complex and multifaceted. It can be driven by underlying health conditions like chronic pain or respiratory disorders, which make it difficult to stay asleep comfortably.

Psychological factors (i.e., anxiety, depression, or trauma) can also be at the root of chronic insomnia, keeping the mind too active to settle into a restful state. Long-standing habits, such as irregular sleep schedules, overuse of stimulants like caffeine, or excessive screen time late at night, can further disrupt the natural sleep-wake cycle and contribute to ongoing sleep problems.

Properly determining whether your insomnia is temporary or permanent can change how you handle it. Short-term insomnia might require relaxation techniques or a few nights of settling into a new routine, while chronic or long-term insomnia might need a more structured approach involving therapy or a deeper dive into underlying health issues.

Despite this, whether short or long-term insomnia, you'll be able to sleep soundly the moment you've tailored your approach to resolve it.

1.3 Other Common Sleep Disorders

While insomnia is one of the more regularly discussed sleep difficulties, there are other sleep disorders that can significantly impact your ability to rest and recharge.

Three of the most common yet often overlooked disorders are restless legs syndrome (RLS), sleep apnea, and sleep paralysis. Understanding these conditions and their symptoms is the first step to finding the solutions to achieve restful sleep.

Restless Legs Syndrome

Restless Legs Syndrome, or RLS, is a neurological disorder that causes an uncontrollable urge to move your legs, especially at night. If you've ever felt a tingling, crawling sensation in your legs that only seems to go away when you move them, you might be dealing with RLS.

This restlessness often flares up in the evening or at bedtime, making it difficult to fall asleep or stay asleep—resulting in broken, fragmented sleep that can leave you feeling tired and drained the next day.

RLS can also worsen with age, and for some, it can become a nightly struggle. The good news is that RLS can often be managed with a combination of simple lifestyle changes and medical treatment. For more severe cases, medications are available that can help regulate the neurological activity contributing to RLS.

Sleep Apnea and Breathing Issues

Sleep Apnea is another common yet often undiagnosed sleep disorder that can severely impact your rest and occurs when your breathing repeatedly stops and starts throughout the night. These pauses in breathing can last anywhere from a few seconds to a minute, preventing your body from getting the deep, restorative sleep it needs.

This sleep disorder often comes with loud snoring, gasping, or choking sounds during the night, and it can lead to daytime fatigue, difficulty concentrating, and even health risks like high blood pressure or heart disease.

These are the two primary types of Sleep Apnea:

- **Obstructive Sleep Apnea**: A more common form of sleep apnea where relaxed throat muscles block the airway.
- **Central Sleep Apnea**: Less common and happens when your brain isn't sending proper signals to the muscles that control your breathing.

Thankfully, just like RLS, sleep apnea is treatable, depending on severity.

One of the most effective treatments for obstructive sleep apnea is the use of a Continuous Positive Airway Pressure machine or CPAP—it's a device that keeps your airway open by providing a constant stream of air through a mask worn over your nose or mouth while you sleep.

Although it may take some getting used to, a CPAP machine can drastically improve your sleep quality and overall health by ensuring you breathe continuously through the night.

Sleep Paralysis

Normally, most people complete their sleep cycle according to the stage—as mentioned earlier in the previous section. However, some may experience a form of sleep interruption during REM sleep, known as sleep paralysis.

Sleep Paralysis is a unique experience where a person, upon waking or falling asleep, is unable to move or speak. It's a temporary immobility, often lasting a few seconds to a couple of minutes—it occurs when the brain awakens from REM sleep but the body remains in a state of paralysis.

During REM sleep, the body naturally undergoes muscle atonia, which prevents the dreamer from physically acting out their dreams. When muscle atonia persists as the brain starts to wake up, it starts up sleep paralysis. Many individuals report feeling pressure on their chest, an inability to breathe freely, and, for some, sensing a malevolent presence in the room.

Experiences such as these can become intensely frightening, though they are not physically harmful. Sleep paralysis is relatively common, with many people experiencing it at least *once* in their lifetime, with some having to experience multiple sleep paralysis states almost randomly. Such sleep disruption is affected by factors like sleep deprivation, irregular sleep schedules, and high stress levels, which can increase the likelihood of experiencing sleep paralysis.

Fortunately, maintaining a regular sleep schedule, reducing stress, and improving sleep hygiene can reduce the frequency of sleep paralysis episodes.

In the event that it *does* happen to you, don't panic. Try focusing on trying to move a small part of the body, like a finger or toe, as these can help break the paralysis. Another way is to force intense movement—jerking, coughing, or twitching helps. If the sleep paralysis continues, focus on taking deep, full breaths to relieve feelings of anxiety.

1.4 Common Causes and Risk Factors

External and internal sleep disruptions are often the problems that are hidden in plain sight in your daily routine. Unpacking the causes and risk factors is the next big step in resolving your sleep problems.

External Sleep Disruptions

Let's start with the most evident causes: caffeine and technology. Sipping on a late afternoon coffee or scrolling through social media before bed can jolt your nervous system into high gear right when you should be winding down. Both of these habits can delay your brain's natural bedtime signals, which keeps you wired when you should be tired.

Then there's the environment you sleep in. When your bedroom is too hot, cold, or noisy—and even the most minor external elements like an uncomfortable mattress or blinding lights—can shift your body out of its comfort zone, making it difficult to stay asleep. Your physical health can heavily affect sleep, too. Sleeping becomes challenging when conditions like chronic pain, asthma, or even allergies keep you up with symptoms like coughing or discomfort.

Internal Sleep Disruptions

Stress is another possible big offender that may cause nightly restlessness. It has a habit of turning your mind into a looping highlight reel of worries at night. Whether it's work stress, personal relationships, or even general anxiety about the day ahead, the tension can keep your body in a heightened state of alertness that's not conducive to sleep.

Even medications for unrelated health issues can also have side effects that disrupt sleep—which, in turn, will cause all of these internal issues to become harder to resolve. All these lifestyle factors round out the list of usual suspects. Irregular sleep schedules, like those caused by shift work or jet lag, can also disrupt your body's internal clock. Even long-standing habits of napping too late in the day or inconsistent bedtime routines can throw off your night's sleep.

1.5 Impact of Poor Sleep on Health

Struggling with poor-quality sleep can feel like more than just waking up on the wrong side of the bed—it can also lead to other internal challenges, such as a weakened immune system and an increased risk of potential mental health issues and possible deterioration.

Physical Toll

Physically, lack of sleep can be highly detrimental to your body, gradually taking a toll on your overall health. Initially, the symptoms may seem minor—a few days of fatigue, headaches, or simply feeling run down. These early warning signs are your body's way of indicating that it's not getting the restorative rest it needs.

Fatigue can affect everything from your focus to your motor skills, making even basic tasks feel more challenging. Headaches often arise from tension and poor sleep quality, while a weakened immune system leaves you more susceptible to catching every cold or flu that passes by.

When sleep deprivation becomes chronic, these issues can compound and intensify.

Compromised Immune System

Without proper sleep, your immune system's effectiveness is compromised, increasing the likelihood of developing infections and making it even more difficult to recover from illnesses.

As a result, you may find yourself experiencing prolonged recovery times or becoming more vulnerable to illnesses that would otherwise be easy to fend off. And it doesn't stop at avoidable issues like fatigue or a simple cold.

Escalated Health Issues

Over time, chronic poor sleep can contribute to serious health problems like diabetes, obesity, and cardiovascular diseases.

These aren't just hypothetical risks; scientific studies have consistently shown the link between poor sleep and these physical health conditions, highlighting the importance of getting enough quality sleep.

Imbalanced Hormone Regulation

Sleep is crucial for regulating various functions in the body, including hormone production. A lack of sleep can negatively influence important hormones like cortisol, leptin, and ghrelin. Elevated cortisol levels, the stress hormone, can contribute to increased blood pressure and cause the body to store fat, particularly around the abdomen. On the other hand, leptin and ghrelin play key roles in regulating hunger and satiety.

When sleep is insufficient, leptin levels decrease, and ghrelin levels increase, resulting in increased hunger and cravings, particularly for high-calorie, sugary foods. This hormonal imbalance can, over time, lead to weight gain, ultimately increasing the risk of obesity.

Impaired Insulin Sensitivity

Another critical area affected by poor sleep is how the body processes glucose. Sleep deprivation can impair insulin sensitivity, leading to an increase in blood sugar levels. This effect can heighten the risk of developing type 2 diabetes, especially if poor sleep is a recurring problem. When the body doesn't properly regulate glucose, it creates a domino effect that impacts energy levels, metabolism, and overall health.

People who experience consistent sleep issues may find themselves in a cycle where low energy levels prompt poor food choices, and disrupted glucose processing worsens their energy fluctuations throughout the day.

Significant Cardiovascular Risk

Cardiovascular health also takes a significant hit from inadequate sleep. During deep sleep, the body's systems undergo important restorative processes, such as reducing blood pressure and allowing the heart to rest. If this restorative phase is consistently disrupted, blood pressure can remain elevated, increasing the strain on the heart and blood vessels.

Over time, this raises the risk of developing hypertension and other cardiovascular issues, such as coronary artery disease. The connection between chronic sleep deprivation and increased inflammation in the body also contributes to cardiovascular risk, as inflammation can damage blood vessels and promote atherosclerosis—the build-up of plaque that restricts blood flow and leads to heart attacks or strokes.

Increased Pain Sensitivity

Furthermore, a lack of sleep can exacerbate chronic pain conditions or create a heightened sensitivity to pain. Without sufficient rest, the body's natural pain regulation mechanisms become less effective, leading to a vicious cycle where pain disrupts sleep, and poor sleep makes the pain worse. This impact can significantly reduce one's quality of life, affecting mobility, productivity, and the ability to engage in daily activities comfortably.

Sleep is more than just rest—it's an essential physiological function that ensures the proper regulation of almost every system in the body, from hormone balance to metabolic function and cardiovascular health. It's during sleep that muscles are repaired, cells are regenerated, and the brain consolidates memory and information from the day.

When the body misses out on these vital restorative processes, it doesn't take long before the consequences start to manifest both physically and mentally. That's why prioritizing sleep isn't a luxury; it's a fundamental necessity for long-term health and well-being.

Ultimately, the effects of prolonged sleep deprivation are cumulative. They may start small, with subtle hints from your body, but over time, they build up and become serious health concerns.

1.6 Common Sleep Myths

Many myths about sleep can actually harm your sleep hygiene instead of helping it. Let's take a moment to debunk some of the most common misconceptions and set the record straight for better sleep.

The Ideal Sleep Duration Myth

One popular myth is that everyone needs exactly eight hours of sleep to function well during their waking hours. While eight hours is often cited as the standard recommendation, the truth is that sleep needs vary from person to person, depending on factors like age, lifestyle, stress levels, and even genetics. For some, seven hours of sleep is enough to feel energetic and focused, while others might require nine or even ten hours to feel fully rested.

It's important to remember that there is no 'one-size-fits-all' when it comes to sleep. What matters most is paying attention to your body and identifying how much sleep you personally need in order to feel alert, productive, and healthy throughout the day. For example, if you find that you naturally wake up feeling refreshed after seven hours, then that might be your ideal sleep duration.

On the other hand, if you feel groggy or unwell even after eight hours, it could mean that you need more sleep or that the quality of your sleep needs improvement.

Sleep requirements can change over time. As we age, the amount of sleep we need may fluctuate. Children and teenagers usually need more sleep than adults due to their growth and development, whereas older adults may find that they sleep a bit less but take daytime naps to supplement their rest.

Factors such as physical activity, illness, and emotional stress can also affect your sleep needs, making it crucial to remain flexible and attentive to your own rhythms.

Rather than rigidly aiming for a fixed number of hours, focus on how you feel during the day. Are you able to concentrate well, manage stress, and maintain energy levels? Or do you find yourself reaching for caffeine, struggling to stay awake, or feeling irritable? These are signs that your sleep might need adjusting.

"Catch-Up Sleep" Myth

You might also have heard that you can make up for missed sleep by sleeping over the weekend. However, the reality is a bit more complicated.

While sleeping in on weekends can help alleviate some of your sleep debt and make you feel temporarily more rested, it doesn't fully reverse the negative effects of not getting enough sleep during the week. The damage done to your mood, memory, and overall health throughout the week can't be magically undone with a couple of extra hours in bed on Saturday and Sunday.

Chronic sleep deprivation takes a cumulative toll on the body, affecting everything from cognitive function to immune system performance, and a weekend of catching up simply can't erase the impact of multiple nights of poor sleep.

Moreover, drastically changing your sleep schedule over the weekend can have unintended consequences, leading to what's often referred to as 'social jet lag.' When you stay up late and sleep in much later than usual on weekends, it throws off your internal clock—much like traveling to a different time zone and then having to quickly readjust. This disruption makes it even harder for your body to get back into a regular sleep rhythm, and it's why you might struggle to wake up on Monday morning or feel groggy and tired throughout the start of the week. Essentially, your body doesn't have enough time to adapt, leading to what feels like a mini case of jet lag.

Instead of relying on weekend sleep marathons, it's far better to aim for a consistent sleep schedule throughout the week by going to bed and waking up at roughly the same time every day—even on weekends. This consistency helps regulate your body's natural sleep-wake cycle, also known as your circadian rhythm, allowing you to fall asleep and wake up feeling completely refreshed and rested.

If you do miss out on sleep during the week, consider taking short naps (no longer than 20–30 minutes) during the day to help recharge, as opposed to drastically altering your sleep schedule.

Chapter 2

Mastering Sleep Hygiene

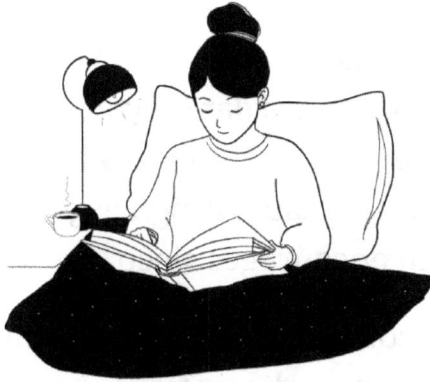

Think of sleep hygiene as crafting the perfect environment and routine to ensure you get the best sleep possible. Setting the stage for a good night's rest, from the comfort of your mattress to the rituals that signal your brain that it's time to power down, are just some of the essentials of your sleep routine.

2.1 Sleep Environment

Having bright lights on or deciding to sleep in a humid bedroom is understandably acceptable for those who grew up in environments with uncontrollable circumstances, such as living in tropical areas or living in a home with thin walls that don't block outside noise that effectively.

However, for others, having an ideal sleep environment is a necessity. It's exactly what you think it is: everything from the lighting to the bedding is set up just right so your body knows it's time to switch off and recharge.

The next sections will provide some insight into the more optimal sleep environment for better sleep.

First, let's talk about your bedroom's atmosphere. It should be calm, quiet, and dark—your cave of comfort. An ideal temperature would be around 65°F (18°C), and a more relaxed room is best because it signals your body to produce melatonin, which encourages sleep.

If any noise becomes an issue, try installing a white noise machine or fan to quiet disruptions. As for light, blackout curtains can be a game changer, especially if you live in a place lit up all night. If blackout curtains are a bit much, however, try contoured or 3D sleep masks that can fit comfortably on your face.

You can also use the type of sleep mask that wraps around your head and secures itself in a way that comfortably hugs your head for a bit of pressure to help settle headaches and migraines.

Next, your mattress and pillows. These are not just about comfort; they're about proper support.

The right mattress should keep your spine aligned and relieve pressure points, while the right pillow should support your neck to prevent cracking and discomfort and not have your head be tilted too far forward or backward from your spine—it's also important that you only use *one* head pillow to prevent stiff necks upon waking up unless you prefer it. Investing in good quality bedding is essential for avoiding painful wakeups.

Lastly, consider the air quality in your room. A stuffy room can hinder your breathing and sleep, and may sometimes cause dried mucus, which can irritate your nose, so maybe crack a window a little if it's not too noisy outside or use an air purifier or air humidifier to moisten the air lightly. Plants can also improve air quality and make your sleep space more inviting.

By tweaking these elements, you can turn your bedroom into a sanctuary for sleep that can immediately convince you to have a restful night. Again, the goal is to create conditions that let your body know it's safe and comfortable to power down for the night.

2.2 Building a Nightly Routine

A good night's sleep starts long before your head hits the pillow; it's about setting the right tone well in advance, much like warming up before a game or tuning an instrument before a concert. Your pre-sleep routine helps prepare your body and mind, signaling, "It's time to wind down and get ready for rest." So, let's walk through what an effective nightly routine might look like.

For starters, timing is everything—try to commit to a regular schedule for sleeping, even on the weekends. This helps regulate your body's circadian rhythm, a biological clock that controls your sleep-wake cycle. When this rhythm gets thrown off too many times, it can make falling asleep and waking up much harder.

About an hour before bed, start dialing down the intensity of your day. Do this by dimming the lights in your living space or switching to lamps instead of overhead lights. This reduces your exposure to bright light—these lights can deceive your brain into thinking it's still day out, thus delaying the production of melatonin, your body's natural sleep-inducing hormone.

Now, let's talk activities. Engage in something relaxing that doesn't involve a screen. Screens must be avoided since the blue light emitted by tablets, phones, and laptops can interfere with melatonin production. Instead, you might want to read a book, listen to soft music, or try easy and gentle yoga stretches. These activities are soothing and can give signals to your body that it's time to slow down.

A warm bath can also do wonders. And no, it's not just about freshening up before bed; a warm bath can raise your body temperature, which may promote drowsiness. Plus, it's a great way to physically and mentally disconnect from the hustle and bustle of your day. Personally, every time I do this, it immediately feels like a natural switch for me to settle down and relax.

Incorporate relaxation techniques into your routine, especially if you find your mind racing with tomorrow's tasks and today's dramas. Conditioning your body with techniques like visualization, progressive muscle relaxation, or deep breathing can also help calm your mind. These practices reduce stress and anxiety, making it easier to fall asleep.

And that's just the activities that we do before bed. As for foods and drinks, heavy meals before bed can often lead to discomfort and indigestion, keeping you up. So, instead of eating dinner later in the evening, try to have dinner earlier in the evening, and if you need a snack closer to bedtime, go for something light and easy to digest.

Avoiding large amounts of liquids right before bed can also reduce the likelihood of nighttime trips to the bathroom. If you want to learn more about the foods that assist you in sleeping a little faster tonight, you can head over to Chapter 4-Nutrition and Sleep.

And then there's the caffeine cut-off. Consider limiting caffeine in the afternoon and evening. Caffeine, on average, can stay in your system for about five to six hours, sometimes longer if you're particularly sensitive to it. So, that late afternoon coffee or energy drink could be a potential culprit if you're tossing and turning at night.

When you're in bed, consider a bedtime ritual that involves some form of meditation or reflective journaling if you're still having trouble falling asleep. This can be a time to jot down what you're grateful for, night-time affirmations, what went well during the day, or even a plan for tackling tomorrow's tasks.

Offloading your thoughts onto paper can prevent them from keeping you awake—just make sure not to overdo it, as you may accidentally stimulate your brain to stay awake and focused.

Creating a nightly routine that promotes good sleep doesn't have to be complicated or rigid. It's about finding what works for you, sticking with it, and making adjustments as your life and needs evolve. The key is consistency and allowing your body to ease into a state of readiness for sleep.

2.3 Sleep Schedule

Getting your sleep schedule locked in will take a bit of practice, a dash of discipline, and a good understanding of your own body's rhythms.

So, why *should* we focus on building a consistent sleep schedule? Well, our bodies thrive on routine.

Maintaining a consistent sleep-wake schedule helps regulate your internal clock or circadian rhythm. Allowing your body to learn when to release those sleep and wake hormones will make the whole process smoother and more natural, which will help you feel less sluggish and more energetic once you wake up.

Let's break down how you can get this right:

1. **Consistency:** First, try to wake up at the same time every day—including weekends. Sleeping in after a late Friday night might be tempting, but varying your wake-up time can throw your internal clock out of whack, much like jet lag does when you cross time zones. A regular wake-up time sets a rhythm that your body can count on, which makes falling asleep at night easier.

2. **Wind-down Rituals:** As mentioned previously, about an hour before bed, start winding down. This means dimming the lights, turning on soft music, or reading a book. This part signals your body that it's time to

shift gears and prepare for sleep. It's the pre-sleep equivalent of cooling down after a workout.

3. **Light Exposure:** Natural light helps regulate your sleep patterns. Try to get plenty of sunlight during the day, especially in the morning. This boosts your vitamin D levels and reinforces your natural circadian rhythms, promoting daytime alertness and sleepiness as night falls. On the other hand, reduce blue light exposure from screens in the evening, as this light can keep you alert and delay melatonin production.

4. **Be Smart About Naps:** Naps are not the enemy, but timing is crucial. Long naps or naps taken too late in the afternoon or early in the evening can mess with your nighttime sleep. If you need to rest and take a short nap, aim for short power naps, around 15-30 minutes, and not too late in the day—think early afternoon at the latest.

5. **Managing Sleep Debt:** If you've had a few late nights, you might be tempted to 'catch up' and sleep over the weekend, but this can disrupt your regular sleep pattern. Instead, try adjusting by going to bed a bit earlier the next night and getting back into your routine as quickly as possible.

6. **Adjusting Your Schedule Gradually:** If your schedule is way off and you want to shift it, do it gradually. Shifting your bedtime and waking hours in 15 to 30-minute increments over several days can help your body adjust without too much stress.

7. **Listen to Your Body:** Finally, pay attention to your body's signals. Feeling sleepy? That's likely your natural sleep window creeping up on you. Try heading to bed when these cues kick in rather than scrolling through social media or binge-watching another episode of your favorite series.

Mastering your sleep schedule isn't just about applying strict rules to yourself; it's about understanding and working with your body's natural rhythms.

2.4 Natural and Artificial Light

Have you ever wondered why camping trips often lead to some of the best night's sleep? Or have you ever wondered why you toss and turn after being on your laptop or phone before bedtime? A lot of that has to do with light—specifically, how it affects your sleep cycles.

Light is like the conductor of your body's biological orchestra, orchestrating the timing of various essential functions, including sleep. As daylight fades, your brain receives the cue to start releasing melatonin, the hormone responsible for inducing sleep. This subtle yet powerful transition signals to your body that it's time to wind down, preparing you for restorative rest.

However, not all types of light are created equal, and the quality of light you're exposed to throughout the day can significantly impact your sleep quality.

Natural Daylight

Natural light during the day is incredibly beneficial for regulating our internal clocks, known as circadian rhythms. Exposure to bright daylight boosts our alertness, energy, and mood, helping us feel more awake and active. Sunlight, in particular, has a unique effect on reinforcing our circadian rhythms, aligning our sleep-wake cycles with the natural rise and set of the sun. This is why spending time outdoors in the morning can be especially helpful for resetting your internal clock—something that can be particularly beneficial for night owls or those struggling with sleep schedule disruptions.

Even just a few minutes of morning sunlight can transmit a powerful signal to your brain that it's time to be alert, setting the tone for the rest of the day.

Artificial Light

Meanwhile, artificial light plays a different tune, one that can often disrupt the harmony of your biological rhythms. The blue light emitted by electronic screens—such as smartphones, tablets, computers, and even some LED lights—mimics the brightness of daytime, tricking your brain into thinking it's still daylight even when night has fallen. This effect suppresses melatonin production, making it much harder for you to fall asleep and reducing the quality of your sleep once you do drift off.

If you've ever found yourself feeling wide awake after watching TV, scrolling through your smartphone, or working on your computer late at night, blue light is likely the culprit. The stimulation from this type of light can delay the onset of sleep, fragmenting your sleep cycles and preventing you from experiencing deep, restorative rest.

Light Exposure Management

So, what can you do to mitigate the effects of light on your sleep? One of the most effective strategies is to maximize your exposure to natural light during the day. Something as simple as taking a short walk outdoors, working near a window, or even opening the curtains to let sunlight flood your space can do wonders for your circadian rhythm. The more exposure you get to natural light during the day, the more your body will understand when it's time to be alert versus when it's time to wind down.

Limiting your screen time before bed is another crucial step you can take to support healthy sleep. Ideally, reducing screen use at least an hour before bedtime can significantly improve melatonin production and help you fall asleep faster. If you absolutely need to use electronic devices in the evening, consider using settings that reduce blue light exposure. Many devices now come with "night mode" or "blue light filter" features, which change the color temperature of the screen to a warmer, amber hue that is less likely to interfere with melatonin production.

There are also apps available that can add a warm overlay to your screen, making late-night device use less disruptive to your sleep.

It's not just about screens, though; the type of lighting in your home also plays a role. Bright, white, or blue-toned lights can have a similar effect to the blue light from screens, signaling to your brain that it's still daytime.

To support your body's natural sleep-wake cycle, consider switching to dim, warm-toned lights in the evening. Using lamps with soft, amber light or even candles can create a calming atmosphere that helps your body gradually transition into sleep mode. Think of it as recreating the effect of a natural sunset—allowing the lighting in your home to become progressively softer and dimmer as bedtime approaches, signaling to your brain that it's time to relax. Creating an environment conducive to sleep involves being mindful of the lighting you're exposed to throughout the entire day.

By intentionally aligning your light exposure with your body's natural rhythms—maximizing natural light during the day and minimizing blue and bright lights at night—you can optimize your sleep quality. This simple yet powerful approach helps you tune your biological clock to the natural rise and set of the sun, setting the stage for a night of deep, rejuvenating sleep. Understanding how light affects your body will give you steps to manage your light environment, which can make a significant difference in how well you rest, helping you wake up feeling refreshed, energized, and ready to take on the day.

2.5 Managing Noise

Blocking out loud noises isn't the only thing that matters when managing noise in your sleeping environment. Sometimes, the right sounds can promote better sleep. This is where the concept of soundscapes and the strategic use of silence comes into play.

For many, the ideal sleeping environment is complete silence, which makes sense because sudden or loud noises can jolt us out of sleep, disrupting the natural sleep cycle.

However, achieving complete silence is only sometimes possible, especially if you live in a busy city, near a busy street, or have noisy neighbors. And when you're used to constant noise, the absence of noise can actually be less soothing than expected. In fact, sudden loud noises can make falling asleep even harder.

This is where soundscapes come in. A soundscape is an environment of sound intentionally created to promote a calming atmosphere. For sleep, these often include natural sounds like the gentle rustling of leaves, a babbling brook, or ocean waves, and yes, including city sounds like a soft, bustling café or low-noise traffic.

The consistent auditory backdrop from these sounds can mask bothersome noises from the environment. The steady, predictable nature of these sounds can be incredibly soothing, making falling and staying asleep easier.

White noise machines are another great choice for creating a beneficial sleep soundscape. They emit a consistent, ambient sound that masks other noises. Whether it's the hum of a fan or the static of a tuned-out radio, white noise provides a continuous sound that helps to minimize the disruption caused by sudden changes in the background noise of your environment.

There are also various apps and devices designed to help create the perfect sleep soundscape. From playlists of calming nature sounds to machines that produce deep, resonant white, brown, pink, or green noise, the options are extensive and can cater to personal preferences and needs.

For some, however, the ideal setup might still be absolute silence. If this sounds like you, consider ways to soundproof your room. This could involve adding thick curtains, sealing gaps in doors and windows, or using sound-absorbing panels on walls. Simple changes like laying a thick rug down can also help absorb sound.

Another technique is to use earplugs, which can be especially helpful when traveling or if you're in situations where you have little control over the external environment. However, it's essential to find earplugs that are comfortable and snug enough to wear all night without causing discomfort.

Managing your sleep soundscape is ultimately about finding what works best for you. It may take a bit of experimentation with different sound combinations and silences to discover what helps you drift off into a deep, uninterrupted sleep.

Chapter 3

Mind-Body Techniques for Better Sleep

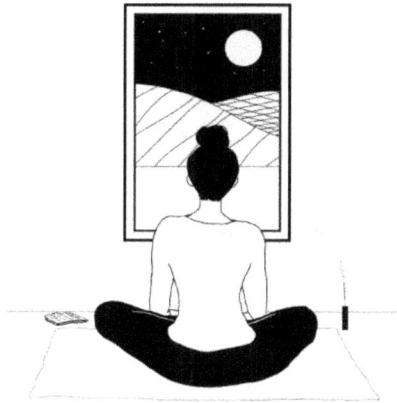

It's time we explore the different mind-body techniques that can positively transform your sleep and boost your overall well-being. From the calming flows of yoga and the self-grounding practice of meditation to the rhythmic ease of deep breathing exercises, these methods combine physical relaxation with mental tranquility, helping you unwind fully at the end of each day.

3.1 Meditation and Breathing

Meditation and breathing exercises work harmoniously together, both involving slowing down, becoming still, and tuning into a deeper part of yourself.

When life's chaos turns sleep into a nightly challenge, these techniques can help you overcome those hurdles, allowing you to drift off into a peaceful sleep.

By incorporating both into your bedtime routine, you can establish a calm state of mind and promote a sense of relaxation that prepares your body for rest.

Mindfulness Meditation

One of the most popular go-to methods for those seeking better sleep is Mindfulness Meditation. This practice encourages you to be present in the moment, observing your thoughts, feelings, and sensations without judgment.

Rather than trying to push away stress or anxious thoughts, mindfulness allows you to acknowledge them and let them pass. Practicing mindfulness before or during bedtime can help quiet the chatter of the day.

Body Scan Meditation

Another helpful technique is Body Scan Meditation, which provides a systematic way to unwind the entire body.

To do this:

1. Start by directing your attention to each part of your body—from your toes and slowly up to your head.

2. As you're focusing on each part of your body, encourage each area to relax and release tension.

This approach can be beneficial if you carry stress in your muscles, allowing your body to let go of discomfort and ease into sleep.

Guided Imagery

Guided imagery involves visualizing calming, peaceful scenes like the slow-moving waves on the shore of a beach or a serene walk in the forest. Here are some detailed steps to do this type of visualized imagery:

1. Find a quiet place, close your eyes, and take a few deep breaths. Focus on relaxing your body from head to toe.

2. Imagine a peaceful scene, engaging all your senses. Picture the sights, sounds, and smells of a beach, forest, or any place where you feel calm and relaxed.

3. Spend a few minutes immersed in your scene. If your mind wanders, gently bring it back. And when you're ready, slowly bring your awareness back to the present, feeling refreshed and calm.

This imagery helps relax both the mind and body, shifting your focus away from stress and creating a positive mental atmosphere where worries are pushed aside.

Mantra Meditation

Mantra meditation is another effective way to calm a restless mind. Silently or loudly repeating a word or phrase creates a rhythm that draws your attention away from distracting thoughts. The repetitive sound serves as an anchor for your mind, fostering a sense of stillness. Whether the word is something simple like "peace" or a traditional mantra like "*om*," focusing on the repetition of words or chanting helps to free the mind from the clutter that can interfere with sleep.

Breathing Exercises

Breathing Exercises are an excellent complement to meditation, helping to regulate your breath and activate your body's natural relaxation response. The science behind breathing exercises lies in their impact on your nervous system.

Focusing on slow, deep breaths tells your body it's time to relax by activating your parasympathetic nervous system (the "calm-down command center") and dialing down the sympathetic nervous system—which controls the fight-or-flight response. This helps to slow your heart rate, relax muscles, and ease your mind into a state of calm.

Diaphragmatic Breathing

Diaphragmatic breathing—or belly breathing—is one of the simplest and most effective techniques. Unlike breathing from the chest, you breathe from right above your stomach.

To practice, follow these steps:

1. Find a comfortable position—whether lying down, sitting, or standing, the key is to feel relaxed.

2. Place one hand on your chest and the other on your belly. This will help you feel the movement of your diaphragm.

3. Breathe in slowly through your nose. Allow your belly to rise more than your chest.

4. Hold your breath briefly, then exhale slowly through your mouth, feeling your belly lower.

5. Repeat for about 10 minutes. You may notice a wave of calmness wash over you after just a few cycles.

4-7-8 Breathing Method

Another powerful technique is the 4-7-8 Method, popularized by Dr. Andrew Weil. This is based on the pranayama breathing exercise that's done during yoga.

This breathing pattern can help lull your body to sleep:

1. Inhale through your nose quietly and softly for 4 seconds.

2. Hold your breath for 7 seconds to allow oxygen to circulate throughout your body.

3. Exhale through your mouth forcefully for 8 seconds, making a soft whooshing sound as you clear out carbon dioxide.

4. Repeat four times, especially before bed, to help calm your mind.

The reason these exercises are so effective is that they focus your mind while relaxing your body—much like meditation.

Instead of letting your thoughts race through the events of the day or worries about tomorrow, you're centering on your breath, anchoring yourself in the present moment. It's a natural way to tune out the noise and tune into a state conducive to sleep.

Including meditation and breathing exercises in your nighttime routine doesn't have to feel like a time-consuming chore; think of it as a pleasant wind-down activity, like listening to soft music or reading a book.

Over time, these practices can cue your body that bedtime is near, helping you create the perfect conditions for a night of deep, restorative sleep.

3.2 Yoga and Stretching

Stretching and yoga before bed can, in fact, improve your sleep. Imagine easing out of your day and into the night with simple stretches that release all that tension you've been carrying around. Doing these routines isn't just improving your flexibility; you're letting your body know it's time to wind down.

Stretching helps in a few ways. It loosens up tight muscles, sure, but it also encourages you to take deeper breaths, which naturally leads to relaxation. You're letting go of the physical and mental tightness that can keep you alert when you should be sleeping at night.

Meanwhile, yoga takes this routine relaxation to another level. It's not just stretching; it combines movements, controlled breathing, and mental focus. This mix is excellent for managing stress and easing the body into a calm state. Even a few simple yoga poses can help settle a busy mind and make it easier to fall asleep. Here are some gentle stretches and yoga poses that are perfect for helping you unwind before bed:

- **Legs-Up-the-Wall Pose (Viparita Karani):** This is one of the best poses for winding down. Just lie on your back, scoot your butt to the wall, and let your legs rest upward against it. This pose is fantastic for relaxing the nervous system and can help if your legs often feel heavy or tired.

- **Seated Forward Bend (Paschimottanasana):** First, sit with your legs straight in front of you. From your hips, slowly bend forward and reach towards your feet. If you can't reach your toes, go as far as is comfortable. This stretch is excellent for letting go of tension in your back and hamstrings.

- **Child's Pose (Balasana):** This pose is a favorite for many – including me. Start by sitting on your heels, then gently bend forward while extending your arms out in front. Let your forehead touch the ground. This is a fantastic pose for soothing the mind and easing tension in the back and shoulders.

- **Cat-Cow Stretch:** Go down on your hands and knees, slowly alternate between arching your back upwards to the ceiling (Cat) and dipping it towards the floor (Cow). This stretch is excellent for the spine and helps bring flexibility to the back, all while deepening your breath and calming the mind.

Adding yoga practices into your nighttime routine can be straightforward; even ten minutes can make a significant difference.

By giving yourself that time to transition from the fast pace of the day to the quiet of the night, you're allowing yourself to wind down and be calmer and more relaxed right before you take a nap or sleep for the day—all while you're building flexibility and mobility into your muscles, as well as helping your body produce dopamine.

3.3 Progressive Muscle Relaxation

Have you ever felt like you're carrying the world's weight on your shoulders? Or notice how your jaw clenches when you're stressed? That physical tension isn't just uncomfortable—it can seriously interfere with your ability to transition into a peaceful sleep. Stress and tension have a way of lingering in the body long after the day is done, creating a barrier between you and a restful night.

This is where Progressive Muscle Relaxation (PMR) can make a real difference. It's a straightforward yet powerful technique to help you shake off the day's stress, release muscle tension, and glide into a more relaxed state, ultimately leading to a night of restorative sleep.

PMR works by systematically tensing and then releasing different muscle groups throughout your body. While it sounds simple, the effects are incredibly profound. When you consciously relax your muscles, it sends a signal to your brain that it's time to slow down and relax as well. This connection between physical and mental relaxation is vital for reducing overall stress and making it easier for your body to prepare for sleep. It is a direct way of telling your brain that you are safe, that the day's pressures can be put aside, and that you can unwind.

The beauty of PMR is that it's not just a technique for easing into sleep—it has numerous other benefits. For one, PMR is highly effective at reducing overall stress and anxiety levels. By regularly practicing PMR, many people find they can manage day-to-day stress more effectively. It's like hitting a "reset" button for your stress levels—a simple and practical way to reset your mental state. Whether it's work worries, personal struggles, or just the ongoing pressures of daily life, PMR can help bring you back to a place of calm.

Another significant benefit of PMR is its impact on managing chronic pain. Tension and chronic pain often go hand-in-hand, creating a vicious cycle where pain leads to tension, which then increases the pain further. By learning to systematically relax your muscles, you may find a decrease in the intensity of pain, allowing for greater comfort and relief. Imagine loosening those tight shoulders or that sore back before you go to bed so they don't keep you awake during the night. PMR offers a gentle, non-invasive way to improve your pain levels and comfort over time.

Additionally, PMR enhances mindfulness and awareness of your body. It encourages you to pay attention to how different parts of your body feel, making you more attuned to areas where tension tends to build up. This increased body awareness is a significant plus for overall mental health, as it encourages you to live in the present and connect with your body's sensations rather than staying in your head, worrying about things you cannot control.

Using PMR before bed is a great way to set the stage for better sleep. It helps turn down the volume on racing thoughts, physical discomfort, and tension that might otherwise keep you awake. Imagine ending your day by lying down, working through a PMR routine, and feeling each part of your body surrender to relaxation—slowly but surely releasing all the stress that may have accumulated throughout the day. It's a gentle invitation for your body to rest.

To get started with PMR, you don't need any special equipment, extensive training, or even a lot of time. You can practice it in bed as part of your wind-down routine— perfect for anyone seeking a simple yet effective way to let go of tension before sleep. Here's a quick rundown to try tonight:

1. **Find a Comfortable Spot**: Lie down in bed or sit comfortably in a chair. Make sure you are in a quiet space where you won't be disturbed.

2. **Start with Your Feet**: Focus your attention on your feet. Tense the muscles in your feet as much as you can—hold for a count of five, and then relax completely. Notice the difference between tension and relaxation.

3. **Move to Your Legs**: Next, move to your lower legs and do the same thing—tense, hold, and release. Feel the muscles loosening as you let go.

4. **Continue Through Your Body**: Gradually work your way up from your legs to your stomach, hands, arms, chest, shoulders, neck, and face. Tense each area for a

few seconds before relaxing. Pay attention to how each part of your body feels after it relaxes.

5. **Take Deep Breaths**: Combine muscle relaxation with deep, slow breaths as you work through your body. Inhale deeply as you tense, and exhale slowly as you let go of the tension.

After a full session of PMR, you may feel a sense of warmth and heaviness in your muscles—clear signs of deep relaxation. Many people report falling asleep faster and even enjoying better sleep quality after incorporating PMR into their nightly routine. You'll feel as though your body is gradually melting into your bed, with each muscle letting go of the tightness it's been holding onto. The real power of PMR lies in its ability to help you relax both physically and mentally. When you practice PMR, you are not just relaxing your body; you are also sending a message to your mind that it is time to let go, to ease away from the day's stresses and worries. You are training your body and mind to recognize the difference between tension and relaxation, which can bring long-term improvements in how you respond to stress.

So, next time you feel wound up before bed or need a practical way to let go of the day's stress, try PMR. It's like hitting a "refresh" button for your entire body and mind—letting go of what's weighing you down, calming your nervous system, and setting you up for a deep, restorative night of sleep.

Chapter 4

Nutrition and Sleep

Understanding how nutrition affects your sleep can be both straightforward and rewarding. The foods and drinks you ingest throughout the day directly impact how easily you fall asleep, how well you stay asleep, and how rested you feel the next morning.

In this chapter, we'll explore how different foods and drinks influence sleep quality, highlighting which can help you sleep better and which might keep you awake.

4.1 Foods That Improve Sleep

Your dinner plate might have more power over your sleep quality than you think. Let's break down some of the best foods known to help you drift off easier and sleep more soundly.

Tryptophan-Rich Foods

Turkey is famous for its role in inducing sleepiness due to the amino acid tryptophan, which helps produce serotonin and melatonin—both crucial for sleep. But turkey isn't the only food that offers these benefits. Chicken, nuts, seeds, and dairy products are also rich in tryptophan and can support better sleep. Adding these foods to your dinner can help create a sleep-promoting environment within your body.

Fruits that Boost Melatonin

Cherries, specifically tart cherries, are one of the few natural sources of melatonin. Simply drinking tart cherry juice or eating cherries can increase melatonin levels and regulate your sleep cycle. Other fruits like pineapple and grapes can also have similar effects, serving as effective alternatives to tart cherries.

Magnesium-Packed Almonds

Almonds are rich in magnesium, which promotes deep, restorative sleep by helping to deactivate adrenaline. Including magnesium-rich foods like these in your diet can reduce nighttime wakefulness and help you relax.

Fatty Fish

Fatty fish, like salmon, trout, and mackerel, are excellent choices for promoting sleep. These contain omega-3 fatty acids and vitamin D, which help enhance serotonin production and regulate sleep. Studies show that eating fatty fish regularly can lead to improved sleep quality and better daytime functioning.

Carbohydrates and Bedtime Snacks

Eating small amounts of whole-grain carbs like oatmeal or whole-grain bread can promote sleep by increasing the availability of tryptophan in the brain.A balanced bedtime snack that pairs a carbohydrate with a protein-rich tryptophan (e.g., an apple with cheese or a banana with almond butter) can support relaxation and make it easier to fall asleep.

4.2 Drinks That Help or Hinder Sleep

When it comes to how beverages affect your sleep, knowing which drinks promote relaxation and which might keep you awake is crucial.

Drinks for Relaxation

Herbal teas, like chamomile and valerian root, have calming effects, making them popular choices for bedtime—chamomile tea contains apigenin, an antioxidant that promotes sleepiness and reduces insomnia, while valerian root tea has soothing attributes that can help you fall asleep faster.

Milk is another sleep-friendly choice, as it contains tryptophan and calcium—both of which help in melatonin production. You could even make "golden milk" by adding turmeric and cinnamon for anti-inflammatory benefits that help your body unwind.

Beverages to Avoid

Caffeine is at the top of the list of drinks that hinder sleep. Found in coffee, energy drinks, and some teas, caffeine can block adenosine—a compound that makes you feel sleepy. Drinking anything caffeinated in the afternoon or evening can lead to trouble falling asleep and disrupt your sleep cycle. Alcohol might make you feel drowsy initially, but it disrupts the sleep cycle, particularly during the second half of the night, reducing overall sleep quality and leading to less restorative rest.

4.3 Timing Nutrient Intake

Timing is everything—especially when it comes to what and when you eat. Eating the right foods at the correct times can significantly impact your sleep quality.

- **Carbohydrates in the Evening**: Consuming complex carbohydrates like oatmeal or whole-grain bread in the evening can help your body utilize tryptophan more effectively, leading to better melatonin production. It's also essential to avoid refined carbs that could spike blood sugar levels, causing disruptions later in the night.

- **Protein Throughout the Day**: Protein, especially tryptophan-rich options like turkey, chicken, and cheese, is best consumed in moderate amounts throughout the day. Combining a protein with a whole-grain carb for dinner or a pre-bedtime snack provides the building blocks for melatonin without overburdening the digestive system.

- **Fats in Moderation**: Fats, while necessary for overall health, can be more challenging to digest. A small amount of healthy fat, like avocado or almond butter, can be helpful before bed, but large amounts of fatty foods might interfere with your ability to get restful sleep.

- **Meal Timing**: Eating your last large meal at least three to four hours before bed allows time for proper digestion, reducing the risk of heartburn and discomfort. If you're hungry before bed, opt for a small, balanced snack to prevent disruptions.

- **Caffeine and Alcohol**: Caffeine should be avoided in the late afternoon and evening due to its long-lasting effects, while alcohol should be limited and consumed earlier in the evening, as it can disrupt sleep patterns.

By focusing on both the type of food and the timing of meals, you can transform your diet into a tool that promotes better sleep.

4.4 Effective Sleep Supplements

When it comes to achieving better sleep, many people turn to supplements to complement their routines. Sleep supplements can be beneficial tools, particularly when used as part of a broader sleep strategy that includes having healthy sleep hygiene and a relaxing bedtime routine. For this section, we'll explore popular sleep supplements, how they work, their benefits, and important considerations to keep in mind.

It is strongly advised to consult with a healthcare provider before starting sleep supplements to ensure that you're using them safely and appropriately for your needs.

Understanding Sleep Supplements

Supplements such as melatonin, magnesium, valerian root, L-theanine, and more can help enhance your sleep quality, but they aren't one-size-fits-all solutions. Each supplement works differently and caters to specific needs, so it's important to understand how each one functions and which might be best for your unique sleep challenges.

Melatonin is one of the most common and well-known sleep supplements available today. It's a hormone naturally produced by your body in response to darkness, helping regulate your sleep-wake cycle. Melatonin is not a sleep inducer but rather a darkness signaler, telling your body it's time to prepare for sleep.

This can be especially useful for people who are struggling with jet lag, adjusting to irregular schedules, or to those trying to reset their sleep habits.

It's important to remember that with melatonin, more isn't necessarily better. Often, lower doses are more effective and can prevent next-day grogginess. While melatonin can work wonders for some people, others may find it less effective.

Magnesium has gained attention as an effective supplement for improving sleep quality. This mineral promotes relaxation and deep, restorative sleep by regulating neurotransmitters like GABA. Magnesium also calms your body down by activating the parasympathetic nervous system, making it easier for you to unwind at night.

There are different kinds of magnesium available, such as magnesium citrate and magnesium glycinate, which are known for being easily absorbed by the body. For those who prefer getting their nutrients from food, magnesium-rich foods include leafy greens, nuts, seeds, and whole grains.

Whether taken as a supplement or incorporated through diet, magnesium's relaxation effects on the muscles and nervous system can contribute significantly to a peaceful night's sleep.

Valerian root, a supplement that has been used for centuries, is used to induce relaxation and promote sleep. Valerian acts somewhat like a sedative on the brain and nervous system, which could help you fall asleep faster with improved sleep quality. However, the effectiveness of valerian can vary widely depending on the product, as supplements aren't as strictly regulated as medications.

If anxiety is keeping you up at night, L-theanine might be a helpful addition to your bedtime routine. L-theanine is a naturally occurring compound, an amino acid, which can be found in teas like matcha, oolong tea, and green tea, and is known for its calming properties. It helps boost levels of calming brain chemicals like GABA without making you feel drowsy, allowing you to fall asleep naturally. L-theanine can be taken as a supplement, or you can opt for a cup of decaffeinated green tea in the evening for a gentle, calming effect.

Another supplement to consider is 5-HTP, which is a precursor to serotonin—a neurotransmitter that can be converted into melatonin. Taking 5-HTP can be helpful for those whose sleep issues are related to low serotonin levels. Typically taken with food in the evening, 5-HTP may support better sleep by naturally enhancing serotonin and melatonin production.

Herbal teas, like chamomile, can be an easy and enjoyable addition to your bedtime routine. Chamomile contains an antioxidant called apigenin, which binds to receptors in your brain that encourage sleepiness and lessen insomnia. While herbal teas may not be as potent as some direct supplements, they can help you relax and signal to your body that it's time to wind down. Valerian root tea, peppermint, and lavender are other popular herbal options known for their soothing effects.

While magnesium can help relax your muscles, pairing it with a consistent bedtime routine that includes mindful breathing can amplify its effects.

Supplements to Avoid Before Bed

While many supplements can enhance sleep, others may have stimulating effects. It's important to be mindful of supplements like vitamin D or certain B vitamins, which may be energizing if taken close to bedtime. Additionally, certain herbal supplements that act as stimulants should be taken earlier in the day. Understanding which supplements work best during the day versus those that help at night will further ensure a peaceful, restorative sleep.

Considerations for Using Sleep Supplements

Sleep supplements, such as melatonin, magnesium, L-theanine, and valerian root, can be effective aids in managing sleep issues. However, it's important to approach them with caution. Not all supplements are created the same, and their effectiveness can vary widely from one individual to another. For instance, melatonin is generally safe but may cause side effects like next-day grogginess if taken in excess. Valerian root, on the other hand, may vary in potency depending on the manufacturer.

It's still best to consult with a healthcare provider before adding supplements to your routine is crucial—especially if you're on other medications or have underlying health conditions, as supplements can clash with certain drugs and may cause adverse reactions. Whether it's using magnesium to relax your muscles, melatonin to regulate your sleep cycle, or chamomile tea to create a calming bedtime ritual, these additions can make a significant difference in sleep quality.

Remember, the goal is to use supplements to support—not substitute—a healthy lifestyle and good sleep habits.

Chapter 5

Natural Herbal Remedies

From age-old herbs of long ago to the modernized natural remedies of today, nature's sleeping aids have always opened up possibilities for improving sleep quality.

You'll discover how these remedies work, the best ways to use them, and the science behind their effectiveness.

5.1 Guidelines for Safe Use of Herbal Remedies

When it comes to getting a good night's sleep, sometimes nature has the best solutions. Natural herbal remedies have been used for centuries to help people relax and get some quality sleep, and these are still commonly used to this day.

Although these types of plants have attributes that have been proven to be highly beneficial in encouraging better sleep and relaxation, it's important to take these natural remedies with safety and careful use in mind.

Here are some tips to safely use herbal sleep aids:

1. **Check with an expert**: Before you start taking natural herbs, discuss with your local healthcare provider for advice. Once you've consulted with an expert, take note of the following:

    a) Take the recommended dosage and check your body for reactions

    b) If you're on medication, ensure that there are no potential interactions.

2. **Monitor Effects**: Keep track of how each herb affects your sleep. Some might work better for you than others.

3. **Consistency**: Give the herb time to work. It might take time to notice a difference.

4. **Quality Matters**: Use high-quality, reputable brands to ensure you get a pure product. Here are some locations you can buy them from:

    a) Grocery and herb stores

    b) Local botanicals

    c) Apothecaries

Not all herbs are best suited for tea, essential oils (for skin, aromatherapy, etc.), or even tinctures—therefore, the following sections will list the more suitable uses of each herb accordingly.

5.2 All-Around Herbs and Uses

Some commonly known herbs have been used in multiple mediums, such as tea and essential oils—whenever applicable.

The following sections are herbs that are proven safe for use.

Chamomile

The first is chamomile. It's one of the most well-known herbal sleep aids. It is mild and generally safe for most people, making it a great starting point if you're new to herbal sleep aids, especially since its gentle, floral aroma can help you unwind.

As mentioned in Chapter 4.2, chamomile has an antioxidant called apigenin—a chemical that helps shut down the forebrain, calming and easing stress tension, which prepares the body for sleep.

Chamomile tea can be prepared and drunk warm 30 minutes before bed to signal your body that it's time to relax. To make this, you can steep high-quality teabags in hot water, not boiling, for about 5-10 minutes.

Chamomile oil can have multiple applications. You can use it in a diffuser or a warm bath for an aromatic pre-sleep ritual or mixed with a carrier oil (e.g., coconut or almond oil) before rubbing and massaging into your skin for additional relaxation. Adding a few drops to your pillowcase to release its calming scent throughout the night is also another good way to use chamomile.

Valerian Root

Next on the list is the valerian root. The valerian root is harvested for medicinal purposes from the valerian plant *Valeriana officinalis*, which is a flowering perennial herb. It's often called nature's Valium—it's been shown to lessen the time needed to fall asleep and improve sleep quality, thanks to how it can increase levels of GABA, a calming neurotransmitter in the brain.

Its strong, earthy flavor, slightly bitter taste, and damp, wood-like aroma can be captivating for many people, though it can be an acquired taste (and scent) for some.

It's generally recommended for short-term use (up to 28 days). So, for best, safe results, it's important to purchase high-quality valerian root to ensure you get a pure product—or opt for valerian root tea bags and essential oils.

Valerian root tea is prepared by steeping a valerian root tea bag for 10-15 minutes. The longer you steep it in boiling water, the stronger the tea and flavor will be. You can elevate the flavor by adding honey or lemon.

A few drops of Valerian root oil in a diffuser or mixing it with any carrier oil and applying this to your wrists and neck can help you de-stress and prepare for the night.

You might consider mixing or blending it with other essential oils, like chamomile or lavender if needed.

Lavender

Lavender is another fantastic and most sought-after herb for sleep. While you might think of it primarily for its lovely scent, lavender has been found to lower heart rate and blood pressure, creating a more relaxed state conducive to sleep.

Lavender tea has a herbaceous and delicate floral flavor with hints of mint and rosemary. Steeping it for 5-10 minutes is ideal. Sipping this tea slowly will allow the calming effects of lavender to help you relax.

Lavender oil, similar to chamomile oil, can be sprinkled on your pillow or added to a diffuser. If you prefer, you can use a dried lavender sachet by your bedside for a more therapeutic bedtime scent. Dilute lavender oil with carrier oil if you wish to apply it directly to your skin.

Lemon Balm

Lemon balm is an excellent herb from the mint family for promoting sleep. It's a mild and sweet herb with a citrusy scent and taste reminiscent of lemons with a hint of mint. It has a mild sedative effect and can help reduce anxiety.

Many people find that a cup of lemon balm tea in the evening helps them unwind and prepare for bed, given its minty and lemony flavor. For lemon balm oil, however, it's not entirely recommended for aromatherapy.

5.3 Herbal Essential Oils

If you're looking for a natural way to enhance your sleep quality, using essential oils is a great option to consider. You can either use essential oils for aromatherapy or apply them to your skin when diluted with carrier oil. This simple and enjoyable practice uses essential oils to encourage relaxation and a restful night. Adding essential oils to your nightly routine can help promote a better sleep-inducing environment for your bedroom.

Aromatherapy

Aromatherapy works by using scents to influence your mood, emotional state, and overall well-being. Essential oils are the key components of this method. These oils, which are concentrated plant extracts, can be used in a variety of ways—whether it's adding a few drops to a diffuser, dabbing some on your pillow, or mixing them with a carrier oil to apply them to your skin safely so you can bring herbal scents with you anywhere you go.

The science behind aromatherapy lies in how our brains process scents—breathing in the fragrance allows the scent molecules to travel through your nose, stimulate the olfactory organs, and send signals to the limbic system in your brain—which regulates emotions, memory, and stress responses.

By using specific essential oils, you can trigger a calming effect, helping your mind and body to unwind and prepare for sleep.

Topical Application of Essential Oils

Applying herbal essential oils to your skin can offer numerous benefits, from promoting relaxation to alleviating physical discomfort.

These oils are highly concentrated extracts that come from plants, and when used properly, they can enhance your overall well-being.

Using herbal essential oils on your skin has its benefits:

- **Targeted relief**: When applied to the skin, essential oils can provide targeted relief for specific areas of discomfort, such as muscle aches, joint pain, and skin conditions.

- **Enhanced absorption**: The skin absorbs essential oils, allowing therapeutic properties to enter the bloodstream and provide systemic effects.

- **Skincare benefits**: Many essential oils have antimicrobial, anti-inflammatory, and antioxidant properties, making them beneficial for maintaining healthy skin.

The effectiveness of essential oils applied to the skin heavily depends on their ability to penetrate the skin's layers and interact with your body. First, there's skin absorption—essential oils are absorbed through the skin's pores and hair follicles, which allows active compounds to enter the bloodstream and apply their effects throughout the body.

Once it's absorbed, cellular interaction happens, where the essential oils interact with the body's cells and begin providing various benefits, such as reducing inflammation, fighting bacteria, and promoting relaxation. However, the *direct* application of essential oils is never advisable. Because herbal essential oils are highly concentrated, you need to dilute them with carrier oils like coconut, almond, or jojoba oil; the usual ratio is 1-2 drops per teaspoon. This ensures safe application and enhances absorption while allowing for an easier, even spread across the skin. Here are some practical tips for topical application to the skin:

- **Dilution**: Prior to skin application, <u>always dilute essential oils with carrier oil</u> to prevent any irritation or adverse reactions.

- **Patch test**: Check for allergic reactions by doing a patch test on a small area of skin before widespread use.

- **Massage**: Incorporate essential oils into massage routines for enhanced relaxation and targeted relief.

- **Skincare routine**: A few drops of essential oil can boost the benefits of your skincare products.

Applying herbal essential oils to your skin is a simple yet effective way to harness the power of nature for improved health and well-being.

Best Herbs for Essential Oils

The list below contains some popular essential oils that are known for their sleep-promoting properties. These can be used for aromatherapy or topical application:

- **Cedarwood oil**: If you prefer earthy, woodsy scents, cedarwood oil might be for you. Cedarwood has a grounding effect that helps ease tension and promotes mental clarity. It is known for calming the nervous system, effectively reducing anxiety, and preparing the mind for sleep. Rubbing this oil on your feet or temples is a good, direct way to achieve a calming effect faster.

- **Bergamot oil**: This citrus essential oil is unique because it can both uplift and calm. Its light, fruity aroma can reduce anxiety and stress levels without being too overpowering. Unlike other citrus oils that can be stimulating, bergamot is especially good for promoting relaxation and improving mood before bedtime. Diffusing bergamot oil in the evening can help create a calm atmosphere and alleviate any pre-sleep jitters.

- **Ylang-ylang oil**: Another excellent option for calming the mind and body, ylang-ylang oil is a sweet, floral-scented extract that has natural sedative properties, helping to slow down your heart rate and reduce blood pressure. These effects are perfect for creating a peaceful transition to sleep. Ylang-ylang oil can be diffused or incorporated into a bathing routine for a more luxurious and calming experience.

- **Frankincense oil**: This essential oil is known for its grounding and balancing properties. It helps reduce anxiety and foster a sense of peace. Its warm, woody aroma has been used in meditation practices for centuries, making it a great option to help quiet the mind before sleep. Applying this to your pulse points can create a sense of calm.

- **Sandalwood oil**: With its rich, woody fragrance, sandalwood is another essential oil that can be highly effective in promoting relaxation. It's known to help quiet an overactive mind and create a sense of tranquility, making it ideal for winding down in the evening.

Be mindful of the quality of the oils you purchase—look for pure, therapeutic-grade oils from reputable and well-known brands to ensure their safety and effectiveness.

5.4 Herbal Tinctures

For this section, we'll focus more on the herbs that can be used as tinctures. Tinctures are another fantastic natural remedy for sleep. Like essential oils, these are concentrated herbal extracts. The main difference is that tinctures are primarily used as medicinal remedies, which you can take orally.

Below are tinctures that may be considered:

- **Ashwagandha tincture**: Often used in Ayurvedic medicine, it is known for its stress-reducing properties. While not directly a sedative, it helps regulate cortisol, which can improve sleep quality.

- **Valerian root tincture**: This is a popular choice for those with trouble falling asleep. It's known for its soothing effects and can help you relax quickly.

- **Passionflower tincture**: This is beneficial for those who struggle with anxiety-induced insomnia, allowing them to relax. GABA levels are increased in the brain.

- **Lemon Balm tincture**: This tea herb works like a mild sedative; it can reduce anxiety and help with sleep.

- **Hops tincture**: One more herb to consider is hops. Yes, the same ones used to brew beer. Hops have natural soothing properties and primarily influence the calming GABA system of the brain—just like the valerian root—unsurprisingly, it's sometimes used alongside this herb because of their similar properties.

Always keep in mind that tinctures are highly potent, so it's better to begin with a small dose to gauge how your body responds and adjust as needed.

Before using tinctures, consult a healthcare professional and carefully review the product labels for recommended dosages. A healthcare provider can also offer insight on potential interactions with other medications or advise if you have underlying health conditions.

Share Your Experience—Make a Difference

Help Others Find Their Restful Nights

> "Sleep is that golden chain
> that ties health and our bodies together."
>
> - Thomas Dekker

When we share, we help others live better. Let's make a difference together! Would you help someone just like you—who wants to sleep peacefully but doesn't know where to begin?

My mission is to make overcoming insomnia and mastering sleep achievable for everyone.

But I need your help to reach more people.

Most readers choose books based on what others say. So, I'm asking you to help another reader by leaving a review of your experience. It costs nothing, takes only a minute, but could transform someone's sleep journey. Your review could help...

...one more parent finally enjoys a full, restful night.
...one more student feels focused and energized.
...one more person finds freedom from restless nights.
...one more tired soul regains their energy.
...one more dream comes true.

To make a difference, simply leave a review.

Thank you from the bottom of my heart for helping others find the rest they deserve.

- *Kiley Manning*

Chapter 6

Cognitive Behavioral
Therapy for Insomnia

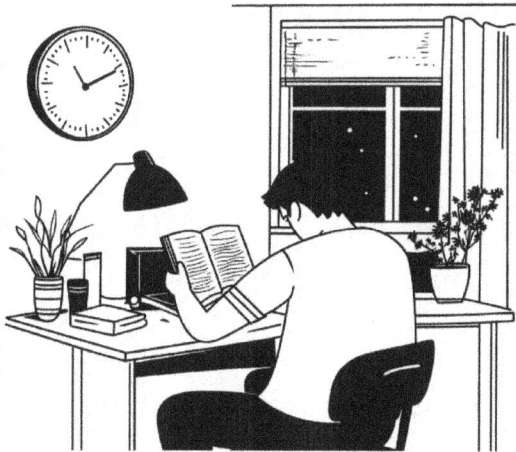

When it comes to tackling insomnia, one of the most effective long-term solutions that have stood out since the 1960s is the Cognitive Behavioral Therapy for Insomnia (CBT-I). Unlike sleeping pills, which can offer a temporary fix but come with the risks of side effects and dependency, CBT-I aims to address the root causes of sleep disturbances by transforming the thoughts and behaviors that interfere with sleep.

This holistic approach to sleep health allows individuals to make sustainable improvements and achieve more consistent, restful nights.

6.1 Core Principles of CBT-I

CBT-I is composed of several core strategies that assist in addressing both the behavioral and cognitive aspects of sleep.

The following are the core components that form the backbone of this system:

Sleep Restriction

Sleep restriction is the first principle of CBT-I and involves limiting the time you spend in bed to the hours you are actually sleeping, which can greatly improve your sleep quality.

When you lie awake for hours in bed, your brain starts associating your bed with wakefulness, anxiety, and frustration rather than rest.

By reducing the time you spend in bed to align closely with your actual sleep time, your brain starts to rebuild the positive association between bed and sleep.

For example, if you're in bed for eight hours but only sleeping five, you limit that time to about five and a half hours, including some time for falling asleep. Gradually, as sleep efficiency improves, you can increase your time in bed, allowing your body to adjust and associate the bed with quality rest.

Stimulus Control

Stimulus control focuses on breaking bad habits that disrupt sleep and reinforcing the connection between the bed and sleep. This means using the bed exclusively for sleep and intimacy—no working, eating, watching TV, or scrolling through your phone.

If you cannot fall asleep within 20 minutes, then you should leave your bed and begin immersing yourself in a relaxing activity, like listening to calm music or reading a book, until you feel sleepy again. Returning to bed only when you feel drowsy helps reinforce the bed–sleep connection, reducing anxiety and frustration.

Cognitive Restructuring

Another critical principle of CBT-I is cognitive restructuring, which aims to identify and challenge the negative thoughts that interfere with sleep. Many people with insomnia experience heightened fears about not getting enough sleep and its potential impact on their daily lives—such as thoughts like "I'll never be able to sleep well again" or "If I don't sleep for eight hours, my entire day will be ruined."

Cognitive restructuring helps replace these anxiety-inducing thoughts with more realistic and positive perspectives. For example, instead of worrying, "I must get eight hours of sleep, or I won't function," you can reframe it as, "Even if I don't sleep perfectly tonight, I can still have a good day." This positive shift in mindset reduces anxiety and helps create a more conducive mental environment for sleep.

Relaxation Techniques

Relaxation techniques are also essential to CBT-I; these reduce your physical and mental tension before bed. It's comprised of techniques such as progressive muscle relaxation, deep breathing, and guided imagery, all of which can help lower stress levels for better sleep.

Deep breathing, for instance, slows your heart rate and relaxes your body, while progressive muscle relaxation involves tensing and releasing muscle groups to transition into a relaxed state.

Guided imagery involves visualizing peaceful and calming scenes—like lying on a quiet beach—to create a soothing atmosphere. Regularly repeating these relaxation techniques can help prepare both the body and mind for sleep, making drifting off easier.

You can return to Chapter 3.1–Meditation and Breathing, to review more relaxation techniques.

Sleep Hygiene

Sleep hygiene may seem basic, but it forms the foundation for healthy sleep. Creating an environment and lifestyle that supports restful sleep involves keeping your bedroom cool, dark, and quiet and minimizing disruptions. You reinforce your body's natural sleep-wake cycle by keeping a regular sleep schedule that requires you to sleep and wake up at the same time every day.

Regular exercise can also improve sleep quality, although it's best to avoid vigorous activities close to bedtime. Steering clear of heavy meals, caffeine, and alcohol in the hours leading up to bedtime also contributes to better rest.

Building good sleep habits ensures that your environment and daily routines support sound sleep rather than disrupt it.

Paradoxical Intention

Paradoxical intention is another technique within the CBT-I toolkit that involves focusing on staying awake rather than pressuring yourself to fall asleep. The idea is to reduce performance anxiety around sleep—worrying about not falling asleep often makes it harder to drift off.

By telling yourself to stay awake, you remove this pressure, and sleep tends to come more naturally. It's a simple yet effective way to break the cycle of stress and sleeplessness.

6.2 Cognitive and Behavioral Techniques

CBT-I isn't an overnight fix but rather a gradual process that addresses the underlying causes of insomnia through sustainable behavioral and cognitive changes.

Sleep restriction and stimulus control work together to rebuild healthy sleep habits by retraining your brain to equate the bed with restful sleep rather than wakefulness. Cognitive restructuring changes the way you think about sleep, helping to eliminate the anxious thoughts that perpetuate sleeplessness.

Incorporating relaxation techniques—such as mindfulness meditation, deep breathing, and progressive muscle relaxation—further aids the sleep process by calming the mind and body. Mindfulness meditation, for example, encourages staying present and observing thoughts without judgment, helping to release worry and stress that might otherwise keep you awake. Visualization, which involves imagining peaceful scenes and engaging all of your senses, creates a calming mental environment that supports sleep.

Writing in a sleep journal before bed can also be effective for clearing the mind of stressors or worries, making it easier to relax and fall asleep.

6.3 Long-Term Improved Sleep Strategies

To apply sleep restriction, start by keeping a sleep diary for one week to record the times you go to bed, wake up, and estimate how many hours you actually sleep.

Based on this data, set a sleep window that matches the time you typically sleep, adding about 30 minutes for falling asleep. Over time, as your sleep efficiency improves, gradually increase the time spent in bed to extend your sleep window while maintaining good quality rest.

For stimulus control, make a habit of going to bed only when you are genuinely sleepy. If you're unable to sleep after 20 minutes, leave the bedroom and do relaxing activities until you feel ready to return to bed. Avoid naps during the day, as they may interfere with your sleep drive at night.

The principles of CBT-I provide a natural, long-term solution to managing insomnia by empowering you to take control of your sleep. By practicing sleep restriction, stimulus control, cognitive restructuring, relaxation techniques, good sleep hygiene, and paradoxical intention, you can effectively retrain your mind and body to sleep well.

These strategies do more than address the symptoms of insomnia; they build a lasting foundation for improved sleep quality.

Whether you've been dealing with insomnia for a short while or for many years, CBT-I can help you break free from the cycle of sleepless nights and empower you to regain control over your sleep health. With commitment and consistency, these techniques can leave you feeling more refreshed, well-rested, and ready to embrace each new day.

Chapter 7

Alternative Sleep Therapies

Alternative therapies consist of effective methods from both modern approaches and also techniques that have been practiced since ancient civilizations.

For Chapter 7, we'll explore these more holistic approaches that offer different pathways, from acupuncture and aromatherapy to sound therapy and biofeedback.

7.1 Acupuncture

Acupuncture might sound a bit intimidating at first, especially if the thought of needles makes you uneasy. But don't let that scare you—this ancient practice has been used for thousands of years to help people relax, heal, and sleep better.

So, what exactly is acupuncture? In simpler terms, it involves inserting thin needles into specific points on your body, called acupoints. These points are believed to be channels where energy, or "Qi" (pronounced "*chee*"), flows.

By stimulating these acupoints, acupuncture helps balance your body's energy and promote natural healing.

Research suggests that acupuncture can be very effective when it comes to improving sleep. One of the ways it works is by regulating the nervous system and increasing melatonin production, which helps control your sleep-wake cycle.

Since melatonin is the hormone responsible for making you feel sleepy, more melatonin often means you'll fall asleep faster and longer. Acupuncture triggers the release of endorphins—natural painkillers and mood boosters—that help reduce anxiety and stress, two of the most common culprits behind insomnia.

Here's what you can expect if you decide to give acupuncture a try. The first step is to meet with a licensed acupuncturist and discuss your sleep issues. They'll ask about your sleep patterns, stress levels, and overall health so that they can tailor a treatment plan to your unique needs. During a session, you'll lie down comfortably, and the acupuncturist will gently insert thin needles into specific points on your body. The experience usually feels like a slight tingling or mild pressure, but it isn't painful.

Once the needles are in place, you'll rest for about 20 to 30 minutes, and many people find this part incredibly relaxing—some even drift off to sleep during the session.

After the resting period, the acupuncturist will carefully remove the needles. Many people report feeling a sense of calm and relaxation afterward, often referred to as the "*post-acupuncture glow.*" This feeling of relaxation can help set the stage for a restful night's sleep.

For some people, the effects of acupuncture are immediate, while for others, improvements in sleep happen gradually over the course of several sessions.

The benefits of acupuncture for sleep are supported by both anecdotal evidence and scientific research. For instance, a study published in the *Journal of Sleep Research* found that acupuncture remarkably improved sleep quality and reduced insomnia symptoms in participants. Another research, which was published in the peer-reviewed medical journal, the *Journal of Alternative and Complementary Medicine,* highlighted acupuncture's potential to enhance both sleep duration and efficiency, making it a promising treatment for those struggling with insomnia.

One of the most compelling aspects of acupuncture is that it's a holistic treatment. It doesn't just target sleep issues; it also aims to improve your overall well-being. By addressing underlying problems like stress, anxiety, and physical pain, acupuncture helps create a more balanced and harmonious state in your body and mind—conditions that naturally support better sleep. For example, if chronic tension or discomfort has been preventing you from relaxing at night, acupuncture's ability to alleviate that pain can lead to better sleep outcomes.

If you're curious about trying acupuncture for sleep, it's important to find a qualified practitioner—someone who is licensed and experienced in treating sleep disorders. Your healthcare provider may have recommendations, or you can search for certified acupuncturists online. A professional acupuncturist will be able to personalize a treatment plan that best suits your needs, helping you not only sleep better but also improve your overall health and vitality.

7.2 Sound Therapy

Music isn't the only sound that can create a calming and relaxing effect on your mind and body. Natural sounds like the gentle rustling of forest leaves, the rhythmic patter of raindrops, or the soft hum of white noise can also help promote a sense of tranquility.

This is the essence of sound therapy, a simple yet powerful method that uses sound to create an environment that contributes to relaxation and sleep. The principle behind sound therapy is that different sounds can influence our brainwaves, nervous system, and overall mood, helping to prepare us for restful sleep.

There are various types of sound therapy, each with its unique benefits:

Ambient Sound Therapy

White noise is one of the most widely used types of sound therapy, and it's often a go-to for those struggling with a noisy sleep environment. White noise consists of a consistent, unchanging sound that masks other disruptive noises, such as traffic, barking dogs, or noisy neighbors. It helps create a steady auditory backdrop that allows your brain to tune out sudden disturbances, making it easier for you to relax and fall asleep. White noise machines are readily available, but you can also find white noise tracks on music streaming platforms and apps, providing a convenient way to block out distractions.

Pink noise is just like white noise but has a slightly different frequency distribution. It features a lower pitch and softer tones, often making it more soothing and calming than traditional white noise. Pink noise is said to resemble the sound of gentle rain or wind rustling through the trees. Research suggests that pink noise may improve sleep quality and memory by promoting deeper, more restful sleep. Its gentler quality can make it an ideal choice if you find white noise a bit too harsh for your liking. Like white noise, pink noise can be found in apps, streaming platforms, and sound machines.

Another variation to consider is brown noise, which has an even deeper frequency than both white and pink noise. Brown noise has a richer, fuller sound, similar to the low roar of thunder or the deep rumble of a waterfall. It's often found to be more soothing for those who prefer a less "hissy" noise compared to white noise. This type of sound therapy can be very effective for drowning out background noise, promoting a sense of calm, and helping you drift into sleep.

Nature Soundscapes

Nature sounds are another fantastic form of sound therapy that many people find incredibly effective. The sounds of ocean waves crashing gently on the shore, a babbling brook, birds chirping, or even the underwater calls of whales can evoke images of tranquil, natural settings. These sounds can trigger feelings of calmness and relaxation, helping you to de-stress and prepare for sleep. Nature sounds are particularly helpful if you feel anxious, as they can mentally transport you to a serene environment. You can find recordings of nature sounds on streaming services, soundscape apps, or even dedicated sound machines.

Sound Wave Therapy

Binaural beats are a fascinating and slightly more complex form of sound therapy. This technique involves playing two slightly different frequencies in each ear, resulting in your brain perceiving a third frequency, or "beat." The frequency of the beat can influence your brainwave activity, promoting a state of relaxation. For sleep, binaural beats typically fall within the delta frequency range, which is associated with deep sleep. This type of sound therapy can reduce stress and anxiety, which allows you to easily drift off into a restful sleep. However, it's important to note that binaural beats require the use of headphones or earbuds, as the effect relies on each ear hearing a different frequency.

Audio Guides

Another effective method of sound therapy is guided meditation or sleep stories. These recordings often combine calming background sounds with a soothing voice that guides you through relaxation exercises or tells a comforting story. The gentle narrative helps divert your mind from stressful thoughts and worries, allowing you to let go of the day's concerns and slip into a peaceful state of mind. Guided meditations and sleep stories are widely available on apps, podcasts, and online resources, specifically designed to help ease you into sleep. Many people find that listening to a sleep story or guided meditation before bed helps them fall asleep quicker and stay asleep longer.

Music Therapy

Music therapy is another great way to enhance sleep quality. With music such as classical, ambient tracks, or even specially composed sleep music, the steady and slow rhythm can aid in lowering your heart rate, relaxing your muscles, and easing your mind into a state of tranquility. The goal of music therapy is to select music that is relaxing but not too stimulating—something that could be played softly in the background as you wind down for bed. It's about finding a sound that resonates with you personally; what might be relaxing for one person could be distracting for another, so experiment with different types of music until you find your ideal match.

Vocal Sound Therapy

Chanting or humming is another unique form of sound therapy that can be surprisingly effective for sleep. Chanting specific syllables, like "*Om*," or simply humming, can help regulate your breathing, promote relaxation, and ease the mind. The vibrations produced by chanting or humming can also create a calming effect that resonates throughout the body, helping to relieve stress and prepare you for sleep. You can find recordings of chants or try practicing them yourself as a part of your bedtime wind-down routine.

Sound Baths

Lastly, we have sound baths, a unique and deeply relaxing experience that combines elements of sound therapy with meditation.

During a sound bath, participants lie down comfortably and are immersed in resonant sounds produced by instruments like singing bowls, gongs, and chimes. The soothing vibrations from these sounds are thought to reduce stress, relax the mind, and promote a deep sense of relaxation—making it easier to fall asleep afterward.

The vibrations from these instruments are believed to influence the brain's frequency, encouraging a shift from the beta state (active thinking) to the alpha or even theta state (relaxation and meditation). This process helps reduce stress and quiet the mind, making it easier to drift into a peaceful sleep.

Whether you're dealing with insomnia or just looking for a way to unwind, sound baths can offer a serene and meditative way to help the mind and body relax.

Incorporating sound therapy into your nightly routine is simple and requires minimal effort. Start by choosing a type of sound that you find soothing—whether it's white noise, nature sounds, or calming music—and play it softly in the background as you prepare for bed. Experiment and try different types of sound to see which works best for you.

Some people find that white noise helps them block out environmental distractions, while others prefer the peacefulness of ocean waves or the guidance of a sleep story.

If you're using a sound machine or an app, consider setting a timer so the sound turns off after you fall asleep, or let it play throughout the night if you find it helpful. You might also explore combining different sounds, such as using gentle music alongside nature sounds, to create a more immersive experience.

7.3 The Role of Technology in Sleep

We often hear about how technology can disrupt sleep, but it can also be an incredible ally in helping us achieve the rest we need. In today's tech-savvy world, there's a gadget or app for almost everything—including improving sleep. Let's explore some of the different technologies that have been developed over the years to enhance sleep.

Sleep-Tracking Apps and Wearable Devices

Tracking apps and devices are some of the more popular tools for understanding and improving sleep quality. Wearables, usually in the form of rings, comfortable wristwatches, or wristbands, can give you a clearer picture of your sleep patterns by monitoring your sleep cycles.

These devices can track how long you're in light, deep, and REM sleep and note how often you wake up throughout the night. Some even monitor heart rate, breathing patterns, and oxygen levels, all of which provide a comprehensive view of your sleep health.

Once you're equipped with this information, you can start identifying and pinpointing factors that may be affecting your sleep. By paying close attention to your sleep data, you can make more informed decisions about your bedtime routine, environment, and overall sleep habits.

Virtual Reality (VR) and Augmented Reality (AR) are two of the most advanced technologies making their way into the sleep health field. Some VR apps offer immersive environments for meditation and relaxation, transporting you to peaceful, calming landscapes—like a serene beach or tranquil forest. These experiences can help you unwind, manage stress, and prepare your mind and body for a night of deep rest. VR relaxation sessions can be especially useful for people who need a complete mental escape from the day's stresses.

In addition to sleep trackers, other wearable technologies have emerged to help promote sleep. Devices like sleep headbands or vibration bracelets use gentle sounds or vibrations to relax you, creating conditions that are conducive to sleep. These wearable technologies work by using biofeedback to guide you into relaxation, helping you transition smoothly from wakefulness to sleep. Some devices also monitor brainwaves and provide gentle auditory feedback to encourage longer periods of deep sleep.

Smart Devices

Traditional alarm clocks often wake you with a loud, jarring noise, which can make getting up an unpleasant experience. Smart alarm clocks, on the other hand, aim to wake you more gently. They use gradual methods like soft sounds, gentle vibrations, or light therapy to ease you out of sleep, often aligning with your natural sleep cycles. Devices like the sunrise alarm clocks simulate a sunrise, slowly increasing the intensity of light in your bedroom to signal to your body that it's time to wake up. This method allows you to wake up more naturally and feel more refreshed in the morning, making the transition from sleep to wakefulness far less shocking to your system.

Temperature is a critical factor in creating the ideal sleep environment. Studies suggest that a cooler room, ideally between 60-67°F (15.5-19.4°C), is best for quality sleep. Smart thermostats allow you to program your home's temperature to automatically lower at bedtime and gradually warm up again in the morning. This ensures that your sleep environment is always at the optimal temperature, promoting deeper, more restful sleep without you having to remember to adjust the thermostat each night.

Lighting also plays an important role in regulating your internal clock, and smart lighting systems like are designed to make this process seamless. These lights can be programmed to simulate natural light patterns, gradually dimming in the evening to signal to your body that it's time to wind down and brightening in the morning to ease you into wakefulness. You can control these lights from your phone, setting them to a calming, warm light in the evening to create a sleep-friendly atmosphere.

Smart mattresses and bedding are also revolutionizing sleep technology. Smart mattresses can monitor your sleep quality and automatically adjust the firmness, temperature, or position to maximize comfort. Some smart mattresses even come with built-in temperature control that cools or warms each side of the bed independently, catering to couples with different sleep temperature preferences.

These innovations allow you to create the perfect sleeping environment tailored specifically to your comfort.

Sound-Related Sleep Devices and Apps

If you're someone who finds it difficult to sleep because of background noise, white noise machines and soundscape apps could be your solution. These devices create a consistent sound—like the hum of a fan, ocean waves, or rain—that can mask loud and disruptive noises, allowing you to relax and fall asleep more easily.

Sleep sound apps offer a wide range of sound options, ranging from white noise, pink noise, and nature sounds, to help establish an environment that promotes a calm and restful atmosphere for sleep.

Many of these apps also feature guided meditations and breathing exercises to further help you unwind at bedtime.

Sleep-Enhancement Apps

The blue light produced by phones, tablets, and computers can hinder melatonin production. Fortunately, many devices now come with built-in blue light filters, which can be scheduled to activate during the late hours of the evening. Screen temperature adjustment programs, or circadian lighting software, can automatically adjust the screen's color temperature, either according to the time of day or however you schedule it, reducing blue light exposure and helping you wind down more effectively.

By filtering out blue light, you reduce its negative impact on sleep, allowing your body to prepare for rest more naturally.

For those who struggle to fall asleep, guided sleep meditation apps can be incredibly helpful. These apps offer multiple varieties of guided meditations specifically designed for sleep, as well as sleep stories that help distract the mind from stressful thoughts. If a racing mind or anxiety keeps you awake, listening to these calming meditations can promote relaxation, making it easier to fall asleep.

Sleep hygiene apps are like having a personal sleep coach in your pocket. These apps provide reminders, tips, and insights on how to improve your sleep habits. They can suggest the best times to go to bed and wake up, remind you to limit caffeine and heavy meals before sleep and help you build a relaxing bedtime routine.

By following these personalized recommendations, you can better maintain good sleep hygiene and maximize your chances of a restful night.

7.4 Exploring Additional Sleep Therapies

The next few alternative sleep therapies in this section are not commonly known and aren't as widely practiced as the ones mentioned in the previous section.

However, they have been gaining popularity due to their unique methods of tackling sleep-related issues.

Acupressure

First, let's talk about acupressure—a practice similar to acupuncture but without the needles. Instead of inserting needles, pressure is applied to specific points on the body to minimize stress and anxiety and promote better sleep.

Like acupuncture, acupressure is centered on the belief that stimulating specific points can help balance the body's energy flow, or "Qi." Some common acupoints for aiding sleep include the space between your eyebrows (often called the "third eye" point) and the spot between your big toe and second toe, known as the "liver point." Applying gentle pressure to these areas for a few minutes before bedtime may help calm your mind and prepare your body for sleep.

To enhance the experience, you can also use acupressure mats and pillows, which are specially designed to stimulate these pressure points while you rest. Lying on an acupressure mat for 10 to 20 minutes before bed can help release muscle tension, reduce stress, and encourage a more relaxed state—creating ideal conditions for sleep. This non-invasive therapy is an accessible option for those who want to explore alternative treatments without the use of needles or medication.

Light Therapy

Another lesser-known approach to improving sleep is light therapy, which can be particularly effective for individuals struggling with Seasonal Affective Disorder (SAD) or irregular sleep schedules. Light therapy uses a specialized lamp or lightbox to emit a bright, artificial light that mimics natural sunlight.

The idea is to use the bright light for a set amount of time each day, usually in the morning, which signals your body that it's time to wake up and be alert.

This exposure helps regulate your body's internal clock, the circadian rhythm, and reinforces a healthy sleep-wake cycle. For those who have difficulty waking up in the morning or experience low energy during the winter months, light therapy can be a game-changer. It's also helpful for individuals who work night shifts or travel frequently, as it helps adjust their circadian rhythm and normalize sleep patterns. Using a lightbox for around 20 to 30 minutes each morning can help improve sleep quality, energy levels, and overall mood.

Biofeedback

Biofeedback is another intriguing method for refining sleep quality, focusing on teaching you how to control physiological functions—like heart rate, muscle tension, and skin temperature—that often affect sleep. During a biofeedback session, sensors are attached to your body, providing real-time feedback on these physical processes. With this information, you can learn techniques to regulate these functions, reduce stress, and achieve a state of relaxation that supports better sleep.

The ultimate goal of biofeedback is to help you become more aware of your body's responses and learn to control them voluntarily. For instance, you may learn how to slow your breathing, lower your heart rate, or relax tense muscles—all of which can contribute to a more restful night. Biofeedback can be done with the assistance of a therapist, but there are also home devices that make it easier to practice on your own. Over time, biofeedback can help you develop better control over the physical factors that disrupt sleep, making it a valuable tool for those dealing with insomnia.

Floating Therapy

Floating therapy, also known as sensory deprivation tanks, is another lesser-known approach that can greatly benefit sleep quality. This therapy involves lying in a tank filled with warm, salty water that keeps you buoyant, creating a feeling of weightlessness. The tank is designed to prevent all external stimuli from entering—such as light, sound, and even the sensation of gravity—creating an environment where your mind and body can truly relax. The weightless sensation helps relieve muscle tension and joint pain, while the complete sensory deprivation encourages the mind to enter a deeply meditative state. Many individuals who use floating therapy report significant reductions in stress and anxiety, which are common barriers to good sleep.

Spending 30 to 60 minutes in a float tank can help you experience a profound sense of calm and relaxation, setting the stage for a better night's sleep.

Yoga Nidra

Yoga Nidra, often referred to as "yogic sleep," is a guided meditation practice that promotes deep relaxation. Unlike traditional yoga, Yoga Nidra doesn't involve physical poses.

Instead, you lie down comfortably while an instructor guides you through a series of body scans, breathing exercises, and visualizations. This practice helps you enter a state of conscious relaxation that is similar to the state between wakefulness and sleep.

Yoga Nidra is especially effective for calming the nervous system, reducing stress, and promoting a restful state— making it easier to both fall asleep and stay asleep. The practice allows you to disengage from the racing thoughts and anxieties that often keep you awake, providing a natural, non-pharmaceutical method for addressing sleep issues.

Many people find that incorporating Yoga Nidra into their bedtime routine helps them achieve more restorative sleep and wake up feeling refreshed.

Chapter 8

Lifestyle Modifications
for Better Sleep

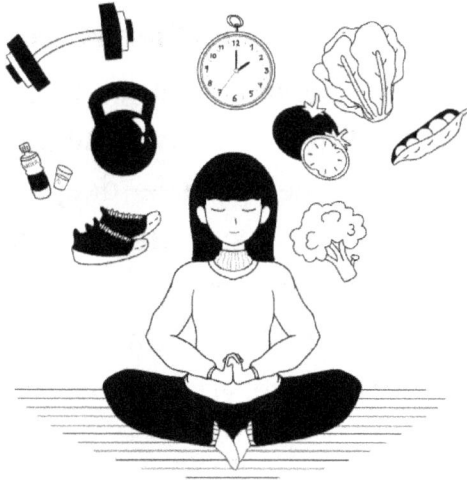

Our sleep quality is greatly impacted by the quality of our lives. The better we manage our waking hours, the more likely we are to rest well at night as well as reap the most benefits out of sleep.

In this chapter, you'll learn about how regular exercise, a balanced diet, stress management, and even the setup of your bedroom can all play a role in helping you get better rest.

8.1 Exercise and Sleep

Exercise, in general, is fantastic for our health. Even better, it's one of the most effective ways to channel excess energy while staying fit. But the connection between exercise and sleep goes beyond just tiring yourself out—regular physical activity can significantly enhance sleep quality and even extend the duration of restful sleep, making it a powerful ally in achieving better rest.

How Exercise Directly Benefits Sleep Quality

When you exercise, several things happen that directly impact sleep quality. Physical activity helps you spend more time in the most vital sleep phase—deep sleep. Deep sleep is where the magic happens: your body repairs muscles, boosts your immune system, and processes the experiences of the day. Essentially, it's like tuning up your engine after a long journey, ensuring everything runs smoothly for the next day.

By increasing the duration of this restorative sleep phase, exercise helps you wake up feeling more refreshed and ready to take on new challenges.

Additionally, exercise helps with regulating body temperature—a crucial factor in falling asleep faster. During a workout, your heart rate rises, and your body heats up. As your heart rate lowers during the post-workout cooldown session, your core body temperature also starts to drop. This gradual decrease in temperature mirrors your body's natural preparation for sleep, helping you fall asleep more easily. When your heart rate drops, blood flow to the skin increases, promoting sweat production, which further cools your body. This cooling effect signals to your brain that it's time to wind down and get some rest.

Timing Your Workouts for Better Sleep

While using up energy and getting in shape are great benefits of exercise, the timing of your workouts plays a crucial role in improving sleep. It's important to know that exercising too close to bedtime can backfire.

Late-night, high-intensity workouts may leave you feeling too energized to sleep. This is because intense exercise stimulates the production of endorphins—natural chemicals that act like a mood booster, similar to the effect of drinking a strong cup of coffee. These endorphins can increase brain activity and make it harder to relax before bedtime.

But if you prefer evening workouts, try to finish them at least one to two hours before you plan to go to sleep. This window allows your endorphin levels to decrease and your body temperature to return to a more natural state, priming you for sleep.

If you're looking to work out closer to bedtime, consider gentler exercises like yoga or stretching that promote relaxation rather than energizing you.

The Psychological Benefits of Exercise for Sleep

Exercise isn't just about tiring out your body; it also has powerful effects on your mental health. Regular physical activity can ease symptoms of anxiety and depression, which are common culprits behind sleep disturbances. When you exercise, your body releases endorphins, which help reduce stress and elevate your mood. This "feel-good" boost can help you go to bed with a clearer, more relaxed mind, making it easier to drift off into a peaceful sleep.

Stress reduction is another significant benefit of exercise that directly impacts sleep quality. By lowering levels of cortisol—the stress hormone—exercise can help you feel calmer as you approach bedtime.

Feeling less anxious and more at peace is a natural prelude to better sleep, and including movement into your daily routine can be a fantastic way to keep stress at bay.

Adapting Exercise to Any Lifestyle

One of the best things about exercise is that its benefits aren't reserved for fitness buffs or gym enthusiasts— anyone can benefit from increased physical activity.

Despite what is commonly believed by most people, you don't have to dedicate hours to intense workouts to see improvements in your sleep.

Even light to moderate activities can make a big difference. Something as simple as a 10-minute walk at a moderate pace every day can significantly improve your sleep quality. Physical activity helps regulate energy, and even short bursts of movement throughout the day can foster better sleep.

If you have a sedentary lifestyle or work a desk job, look for ways to add a little more movement to your day. For example, you could stand up every hour for a quick stretch, do a few squats, or try some wall push-ups. You can also take short walks around your workspace during breaks. These small efforts, though seemingly minimal, can collectively enhance your ability to rest at night.

For those who have time for more regular exercise, consider engaging in rhythmic, aerobic activities like swimming, cycling, or brisk walking. These types of exercises can help elevate your heart rate and are particularly effective for deepening sleep. If stress is a major factor that interferes with your sleep, incorporating yoga or Pilates can be incredibly beneficial.

These practices combine physical activity with mindfulness and relaxation techniques, helping you unwind both physically and mentally.

Making Exercise a Sustainable Part of Your Routine

Optimizing exercise for better sleep isn't about making monumental lifestyle changes; it's more about finding enjoyable ways to add movement to your day. This means prioritizing activities that fit into your lifestyle and that you can see yourself sticking with long-term. Whether it's a morning yoga session, a lunchtime walk, or a few minutes of stretching before bed, making exercise a regular habit can transform your sleep quality over time.

It's important to remember that exercise isn't just a tool for better sleep—it's a key element in leading a healthy and fulfilling lifestyle. The better you sleep, the more energy and motivation you'll have for your workouts, and the more you exercise, the better you'll sleep.

Incorporating this positive cycle can enrich both your waking and resting hours, helping you feel your best throughout the day and promoting deep, restorative rest at night.

8.2 Alcohol and Caffeine Intake

Late-night coffee or a couple of beers at home might seem like a relaxing way to wind down, but they can seriously disrupt your sleep.

Let's explore why alcohol and caffeine aren't effective sleep aids and how they can actually work against your rest.

Caffeinated Drinks

It's no secret that caffeine is a powerful stimulant—it's known to increase alertness, boost energy, and improve focus. However, it also works against the processes that help you fall asleep. The issue lies in caffeine's long half-life, which is about 5 to 6 hours on average. If you drink a cup of coffee at 4 p.m., about half of that caffeine is still active in your system by 10 p.m., keeping you wired just when you need to wind down.

Caffeine works by blocking adenosine, a natural brain chemical that makes you feel sleepy as it accumulates throughout the day. When caffeine prevents adenosine from binding to its receptors, it tricks your brain into feeling more alert, delaying your body's natural sleep signals. It's also important to consider that caffeine isn't just hiding in coffee. It also sneaks into less obvious places like tea, chocolate, and even some pain relievers and weight loss pills.

So, that late-night chocolate snack or over-the-counter headache medicine might unintentionally keep you up, even if you haven't had a cup of coffee in hours.

Because of caffeine's long-lasting effects, consuming it late in the day will make it more difficult for you to fall asleep, experience lighter sleep, and have frequent awakenings throughout the night.

Alcoholic Beverages

Alcohol is another common substance that often gets mistaken for a sleep aid. A nightcap may help you feel drowsy, making it easier to fall asleep, but the sedative effect of alcohol is misleading when it comes to sleep quality.

This disrupts your REM sleep—the stage of sleep that's essential for dreaming and cognitive processing.

REM sleep manages memory consolidation, emotional regulation, and overall mental health. When alcohol reduces REM sleep, it prevents you from getting the restorative benefits of this crucial sleep phase, leading to poor-quality sleep.

The result? You might fall asleep quickly, but you end up in a less restorative sleep and often wake up feeling groggy and unrested.

Another issue with alcohol is that it's a diuretic—which means it increases urine production. You might have noticed needing to run to the bathroom more often after a few drinks, and this doesn't stop when you fall asleep.

Instead, it increases your chances of waking up in the middle of the night to use the bathroom. These interruptions further compromise your sleep quality, leading to more fragmented and less satisfying rest.

How to Manage Caffeine and Alcohol

It's a good idea to limit caffeine consumption to the morning or early afternoon. As a rule of thumb, it's best to avoid caffeine after 2 p.m.—this will give your body enough time to process and clear it from your system well before bedtime. This way, caffeine's stimulating effects won't interfere with your natural sleep signals, allowing you to wind down properly at night.

Alcohol is also best consumed in moderation. If you enjoy a drink in the evening, try to have it earlier—ideally three to four hours before bedtime—and limit yourself to one or two drinks. This allows your body more time to metabolize the alcohol before you go to sleep, reducing its impact on your sleep cycle. Drinking water alongside alcoholic beverages can also help reduce the dehydration that often accompanies alcohol, which can disrupt sleep even further.

Staying hydrated by regularly reminding yourself to drink water can mitigate some of the negative effects and may reduce the likelihood of waking up at night.

Individual Sensitivities and Tracking Habits

It's worth noting that different people have different levels of sensitivity to caffeine and alcohol. Genetics and metabolism play a large role in how quickly your body processes these substances, and you may notice that some people can drink coffee late in the day without any trouble while others might be affected by even small amounts.

Similarly, while some people can tolerate a glass of wine without experiencing any significant sleep disruptions, others find it significantly interferes with their sleep. Because everyone is different, keeping track of your sleep habits in a sleep diary can be incredibly helpful.

Write down what time you consumed caffeine or alcohol, how much you had, and how it seemed to impact your sleep that night. By doing this consistently, you can start to see patterns and make informed decisions about the timing and amounts of these substances that work best for you.

For example, you might notice that even a small amount of caffeine after lunch disrupts your sleep or that you need to finish your evening glass of wine by 7 p.m. to avoid waking up during the night. Caffeine and alcohol can both significantly affect your sleep quality, but managing their impact is all about timing and moderation.

By understanding how these substances affect your body and adjusting your habits accordingly, you can ensure that they don't stand in the way of a restful night's sleep.

8.3 Stress Management

Stress is one of the most common and disruptive obstacles to a good night's sleep. When stress strikes, it triggers your body's "fight or flight" response, releasing hormones like cortisol and adrenaline to keep you on high alert.

While this response is incredibly useful if you're in immediate danger—like our ancestors facing wild animals—it's much less helpful when your stressors are modern-day issues like work deadlines, family conflicts, or financial worries. These aren't situations in which you can simply "fight" or "flee," and the prolonged activation of this stress response can make it nearly impossible to relax and fall asleep.

The fight-or-flight response prepares your body to take action, raising your heart rate, increasing blood pressure, and tightening your muscles—the opposite of what your body needs to drift into a peaceful sleep. Chronic stress means your body is perpetually on high alert, unable to enter the rest-and-digest state.

Essentially, it's like having an emergency alarm constantly ringing in the background, preventing you from winding down when it's time for bed.

Prolonged stress can also lead to racing thoughts. Imagine yourself lying in bed, staring at the ceiling, replaying every conversation, worrying about tomorrow's to-do list, or rehashing past mistakes. This constant mental chatter keeps your brain engaged and alert, making it difficult to go to sleep, stay asleep, or enter deeper stages of sleep. The more you worry about not sleeping, the more stressed you become, leading to a vicious cycle of stress-induced insomnia.

The effects of stress on sleep go beyond just difficulty falling asleep. Stress can heavily impact the quality of your sleep, preventing you from reaching the deeper, restorative stages like slow-wave sleep (deep sleep) and REM sleep. These are the sleep stages where your body repairs itself, consolidates memories, and processes emotions. When stress keeps you in a state of shallow sleep, you miss out on these benefits, leading to fatigue, impaired focus, and emotional instability the next day.

Furthermore, cortisol, often referred to as the stress hormone, is particularly problematic when it comes to sleep. Normally, cortisol levels decrease in the evening, allowing your body to relax.

However, when you're stressed, cortisol levels remain elevated well into the night, making it difficult for your body to recognize it's time to sleep. This high cortisol level can lead to fragmented sleep, making you more likely to wake up frequently and struggle to return to sleep.

8.4 Social Connections and Sleep

Sleep is influenced not only by your diet and lifestyle but also by the quality of your social connections. Strong relationships play an essential role in supporting healthy sleep, as humans, even those who are introverted, need social interaction. Nurturing meaningful connections can significantly improve your ability to rest well each night.

Having good and healthy relations with the people close to you can create a great web of connections that can act as a secure and comfortable blanket when faced with stressors and problems. A good circle of trustworthy friends, for example, can provide support for day-to-day stresses that keep you up at night.

Humans, being social creatures by nature, need strong connections to release neurotransmitters like oxytocin — the "love hormone" that relieves stress and makes you feel secure and content.

Healthy relationships give a sense of security and belonging, making the world feel less overwhelming. Knowing that there's someone you can rely on can greatly reduce the anxiety and worries that often keep us awake at night. Even talking to a friend can sometimes feel like a weight has been lifted off your shoulders—it's not just an emotional release; it's also fostering great sleep.

On the other hand, feeling isolated or having strained relationships can crank up your stress levels and lead to depression and anxiety, which are all notorious sleep stealers. Stress about relationships can trigger the body's fight or flight response, releasing cortisol, which can keep you alert and awake when you should be winding down.

Try bolstering your social connections if you want to improve your sleep quality.

Here are a few tips:

- **Reach Out Regularly**: Keeping in touch is easier than ever in the digital age. A text, a call, or even a comment on a social media post can strengthen bonds, whether it's with family, old friends, or new acquaintances.

- **Be Present**: Give them your full attention when you're with someone. Being present makes interactions more meaningful and deepens connections, enhancing that comforting social blanket.

- **Join Groups or Clubs**: Engaging in social activities can expand your social network and fill your calendar with enjoyable outings that boost your mood and help you feel connected.

- **Volunteer**: Helping others is a fantastic way to connect with people and improve your emotional well-being, which is excellent for sleep.

- **Resolve Conflicts**: This might be challenging, but addressing and resolving interpersonal conflicts can significantly reduce stress. Sometimes, simply agreeing to disagree can bring a sense of peace, helping to ease your mind and improve your sleep.

- **Share Your Feelings**: Opening up about your thoughts and feelings can deepen your relationships and alleviate stress. It's okay to be vulnerable; you'll often find others facing similar struggles.

- **Ask for Help**: If you're feeling down or overwhelmed, reach out for support. It's not a sign of weakness but a step toward building more robust, supportive relationships.

- **Pet Ownership**: Having an animal friend can also increase oxytocin and lower cortisol. Caring and spending time with them can improve your well-being, which, in turn, enhances your sleep quality. The feelings of social isolation significantly decrease when you're spending time with your beloved pets, whether they're furry, feathered, or even have scales.

Cultivating solid social ties can create a supportive environment that enhances sleep quality. Your social life should be a source of comfort, not stress. So, nurture those connections—it's good for your social life, sleep, and overall health.

Chapter 9

Special Considerations and Populations

While sleep is a universal need, how we experience and achieve it differs greatly across life stages, genders, and unique circumstances like shift work or frequent travel. These variations bring unique challenges that require tailored approaches to support optimal rest and well-being.

In this chapter, we'll explore the specific needs of different groups, considering factors such as age, lifestyle, and health conditions, and provide practical strategies to help each find their path to better sleep.

9.1 Sleep Challenges Across Life Stages

From newborns to seniors, the sleep challenges we face change as our bodies and lifestyles shift, requiring unique approaches to address each phase effectively.

Newborns and Infants

Newborns and infants follow a sleep schedule that may seem unpredictable and fragmented from an adult's perspective.

Typically, babies sleep 16 to 17 hours a day, but this sleep is spread across multiple short periods throughout both day and night. This irregular pattern occurs because their circadian rhythms are still developing and don't fully mature until around 3 to 6 months of age. For parents, this often means frequent nighttime awakenings and a sleep routine that shifts as the baby grows.

While this phase can be challenging, there are ways to gently guide your baby toward healthier sleep habits.

Introducing a consistent bedtime routine, such as a warm bath, soft lullabies, or gentle rocking, helps signal to your baby that it's time to wind down. Creating a calm and dimly lit environment during nighttime feedings and diaper changes can also reinforce the distinction between day and night.

As babies grow and their biological clocks mature, these early routines help establish a more predictable sleep pattern. By around three months of age, many infants start to consolidate sleep into longer stretches at night, giving parents a glimpse of relief and setting the stage for a more stable sleep schedule.

It may feel exhausting at first, but these gradual adjustments and habits play a fundamental role in supporting your baby's sleep development and overall well-being.

Toddlers and Preschoolers

As infants transition into toddlers and preschoolers, their sleep challenges evolve, often revolving around bedtime resistance, nighttime fears, and the influence of modern technology. Toddlers frequently test boundaries by refusing to go to bed, delaying sleep with endless requests, or seeking repeated reassurance from caregivers. This developmental stage is also marked by the emergence of fears, such as being afraid of the dark or experiencing nightmares, which can make bedtime an emotionally charged experience for both the child and the parents.

In recent years, an additional modern challenge has emerged: increased screen time among toddlers and preschoolers.

Devices like tablets and smartphones, while sometimes helpful for entertainment or learning, can inadvertently disrupt sleep patterns. The blue light emitted by screens inhibits melatonin production. This can delay sleep onset and lead to fragmented or poor-quality sleep.

Moreover, prolonged exposure to screens may contribute to issues like inattention, overstimulation, and difficulty winding down before bed. Establishing a comforting and predictable bedtime routine is one of the most effective ways to address these challenges.

Activities like reading a bedtime story, having a warm drink, or engaging in gentle snuggles can create a positive association with sleep. Including a soft nightlight can help ease fears of the dark while ensuring the room environment is calm and conducive to rest.

Keeping an easy-to-follow bedtime routine consistent is essential for your toddler's growth. Having the same calming steps each night helps signal to the child that it's time to sleep.

To combat the impact of screen time, it's essential to set firm boundaries around device use:

- **Under 2 years old**: Avoid screen time entirely, except for video chatting with family or friends to maintain social connections.
- **Ages 2-5 years**: Limit screen time to no more than one hour per day of high-quality programming, ideally co-viewed with a parent or sibling to encourage interaction and discussion.

Incorporating device-free periods, especially in the hour before bedtime, can significantly improve sleep quality. Encourage alternative calming activities, like playing with toys, engaging in quiet family interactions, or enjoying a soothing bath.

By setting clear boundaries, fostering healthy sleep routines, and managing screen time effectively, parents can help their toddlers and preschoolers overcome these common sleep hurdles and develop habits that support better rest and overall well-being.

School-Age Children

School-age children, ranging from ages 5 to 12, encounter unique sleep challenges as they navigate a more structured and demanding phase of life. Increased academic pressures, busy extracurricular schedules, and expanding social obligations can make it difficult to prioritize consistent bedtimes.

Other factors that may also add another layer of complexity for these children would be increased anxiety relating to school performance, friendships, or upcoming events, which would cause restlessness or difficulty falling asleep.

This stage is also marked by greater independence, which can lead to bedtime resistance or a desire to stay up later. Peer influences and access to technology, such as video games, smartphones, and televisions, can further interfere with their ability to wind down before bed. The blue light emitted by screens suppresses melatonin production, delaying the body's natural sleep onset.

Children in this age group typically require 9 to 12 hours of sleep per night to support their physical growth, cognitive development, and emotional well-being.

Lack of adequate sleep can lead to issues such as reduced focus, irritability, weakened immune function, and poor academic performance. Forming and maintaining consistent sleep patterns is critical to ensuring they get the rest their developing bodies and minds need.

Teenagers

As children transition into their teenage years, their sleep needs and schedules shift dramatically. Adolescence brings a biological change known as a *delayed sleep phase*, where the body's natural circadian rhythm prompts teens to stay awake later and wake up later.

This is driven by changes in melatonin production, which is released later at night during puberty.

While teens still require 8-10 hours of sleep per night to support their growth, brain development, and emotional regulation, early school start times and busy schedules often make achieving this goal difficult, leading to chronic sleep deprivation.

Below are common sleep challenges that teens face:

1. **Biological Changes:** The delayed sleep phase causes teens to naturally feel tired later in the evening, but this conflicts with early morning wake-up times for school. This mismatch between biological needs and societal demands often leads to insufficient sleep during the week, with many teens attempting to "catch up" by sleeping in on weekends, further disrupting their circadian rhythm.

2. **Academic and Extracurricular Pressures:** Teens face increasing demands from schoolwork, sports, clubs, and part-time jobs, all of which can encroach on their sleep time. Late-night study sessions or after-school activities can push bedtimes even later.

3. **Digital Distractions:** Smartphones, tablets, gaming consoles, and other electronic devices often keep teens awake into the late hours. The blue light emitted from screens suppresses melatonin production, further delaying sleep onset, while social media and online interactions can be mentally stimulating, making it harder to unwind.

4. **Social Priorities:** Adolescents often prioritize socializing, oversleeping, staying up late to chat with friends, attending events, or participating in online activities. Peer pressure and the fear of missing out (FOMO) can lead teens to sacrifice sleep for social engagement.

It's important to approach sleep challenges with empathy and understanding. Rather than imposing strict rules, collaborate with teens to develop routines that prioritize sleep while respecting their autonomy.

Frame good sleep habits as a tool for achieving their goals—whether excelling in school, performing well in sports, or maintaining friendships. By encouraging teens to view sleep as a vital component of their health and success, you can help them build habits that will not only benefit them during adolescence but also lay the foundation for a lifetime of better sleep and well-being.

Adults

Adults are certainly not exempt from sleep challenges. Work demands, family responsibilities, and caregiving duties, whether for children or aging parents, can make it challenging to get enough quality sleep. Adults are more susceptible to insomnia, which can be triggered by stress, anxiety, or a constantly changing schedule.

Sleep issues like sleep apnea are also more common in this stage of life, particularly for those who struggle with weight gain or other health concerns. Adults can benefit from prioritizing a consistent sleep schedule, which means planning out when they go to bed and wake up at the same time every day, even on weekends.

Creating a relaxing pre-sleep routine—whether it's reading a book, practicing yoga, or engaging in mindful breathing exercises—can be an effective way to signal to the body that it's time to wind down and rest.

Older Adults and Seniors

As people age, sleep patterns often shift, leading to challenges that many assume are just part of getting older. However, these difficulties—such as trouble falling asleep, staying asleep, or waking up too early—are often influenced by factors beyond age itself.

Health issues like arthritis, chronic pain, heart disease, or conditions such as sleep apnea can play a significant role. Additionally, certain medications prescribed for age-related health concerns may disrupt natural sleep cycles. Reduced physical activity and changes in the body's internal clock can further contribute to fragmented sleep.

Older adults are also more likely to wake multiple times during the night and may spend less time in restorative deep sleep phases, leading to feelings of fatigue or grogginess in the morning. Over time, these disruptions can affect mood, cognitive function, and overall quality of life. Addressing these challenges starts with creating a sleep-friendly environment. A cool, dark, and quiet bedroom is essential for promoting restful sleep.

Simple lifestyle adjustments, such as limiting caffeine and alcohol intake in the afternoon, managing stress through relaxation techniques, and incorporating light physical activity like walking or yoga during the day, can also make a significant difference. Additionally, consulting a doctor to manage underlying health conditions and discussing alternatives for sleep-disrupting medications can provide targeted relief. Understanding and addressing these challenges is not just about improving sleep—it's about enhancing overall well-being.

Recognizing that sleep difficulties in older adults are not inevitable opens the door to solutions that support healthier, more restorative rest. By empathizing with and supporting others through their unique sleep challenges— whether it's a toddler navigating fears, a teen adjusting to biological shifts, or an older adult facing health-related disruptions—we foster an environment of understanding and care across all life stages.

9.2 Gender-Specific Sleep Issues

Sleep affects everyone differently, especially when it comes to gender differences. Men and women can face distinct challenges when trying to get a good night's rest. Taking the time to understand these challenges can help you identify the root of your own sleep difficulties or those of your loved ones, making it easier to find effective solutions.

Sleep Issues in Women

For many women, several health and gender-specific issues can interrupt their normal sleep schedule. These disturbances are often linked to the unique physiological processes that women experience throughout their lives.

Here are some women-specific issues that can interrupt the flow of their sleep:

- **Hormonal Fluctuations**: Hormonal changes can drastically affect how well women sleep. During their menstrual cycle, the rise and fall of estrogen and progesterone can often interrupt sleep patterns, leading to difficulty falling asleep, staying asleep, or feeling rested upon waking. Women may also experience premenstrual symptoms such as cramps, bloating, and mood swings, further contributing to sleep disturbances.

- **Pregnancy**: Pregnancy brings its own unique challenges, especially in the later stages. Physical discomfort from a growing belly, leg cramps, back pain, and continual trips to the bathroom all make the usual comfortable sleeping positions feel awkward, as well as increased difficulty in staying asleep throughout the night. Additionally, anxiety about the upcoming birth and changes in lifestyle can keep expectant mothers awake. After giving birth, new mothers face a different set of challenges, as they must adjust their sleep schedules to match the erratic patterns of their newborns, which can leave them feeling perpetually exhausted.

- **Menopause**: Menopause is another pivotal time for sleep disruptions in women. Hot flashes and night sweats are some of the common symptoms that wake women up multiple times throughout the night, often leaving them drenched and uncomfortable. Decreased estrogen levels can also make it more exhausting for women when it comes to falling and staying asleep. The constant sleep disturbances that occur during menopause can significantly impact daily functioning and overall well-being. Strategies such as maintaining a cool and calming sleep environment, practicing relaxation techniques, and possibly exploring hormone replacement therapy (HRT) with a doctor can help manage these symptoms and improve sleep quality.

Sleep Issues in Men

Men, on the other hand, often face sleep issues related to specific health conditions that become more prevalent as they age. These challenges can greatly impact their quality of sleep and overall health.

Some men-specific sleep issues that can disrupt sleep can include:

- **Sleep Apnea**: Obstructive sleep apnea (OSA) is statistically more common and often more severe in men than in women. This disorder involves frequent interruptions in breathing during sleep, leading to fragmented, non-restorative sleep and excessive daytime sleepiness. The condition is often linked to obesity, smoking, and alcohol consumption—all factors that can exacerbate sleep apnea symptoms. If left untreated, sleep apnea can heighten the probability of developing cardiovascular disease and other health issues. Seeking treatment, such as using a continuous positive airway pressure (CPAP) machine, can help alleviate symptoms and improve sleep quality.

- **Erectile Dysfunction (ED):** At around the age of 40, around 40% of men may begin to experience some degree of erectile dysfunction, and this occurrence becomes even more common as they reach their 70s. ED can often be linked to other health issues like cardiovascular disease, obesity, hormonal imbalances, and psychological factors such as anxiety and depression. The stress and emotional burden that accompany ED can significantly disrupt sleep, contributing to a vicious cycle of sleeplessness and mental strain. Addressing these underlying health concerns can help improve both ED and sleep quality.

- **Prostate Issues:** Several common prostate issues in men can disrupt sleep. Around the age of 60, many men experience benign prostatic hyperplasia (BPH), a non-cancerous enlargement of the prostate gland. This condition often causes frequent nighttime urination, leading to multiple awakenings throughout the night and reduced sleep quality. Additionally, prostatitis, an inflammation of the prostate, affects about 5-10% of young and middle-aged men. This condition can cause pain and discomfort, further interfering with sleep. Medical treatment and lifestyle changes, such as reducing fluid intake in the evening, can help manage symptoms and improve sleep.

- **Hormonal Imbalance**: Hormonal fluctuations are not exclusive to women. As men age, typically starting in their 30s, some may begin to experience low testosterone levels. Low testosterone can contribute to increased health risks, including obesity, cardiovascular diseases, and chronic fatigue. The cycle of exhaustion and poor sleep that follows can perpetuate further fatigue, making it essential to address hormonal imbalances through lifestyle modifications or hormone therapy.

- **Cardiovascular Disease**: Men have an increased risk of developing heart disease as they age, especially if they engage in unhealthy lifestyle habits like poor diet, lack of exercise, and smoking. Cardiovascular disease can lead to sleep disruptions, particularly if associated with conditions like restless leg syndrome (RLS), which is more prevalent in men with poor cardiovascular health. Addressing underlying heart issues by adopting a heart-healthy diet and consistently engaging in physical activity can help improve sleep quality and overall well-being.

Men and women can benefit greatly from maintaining a healthier lifestyle, with regular exercise and a consistent sleep schedule in a bedroom that's put together with sleep hygiene in mind. However, addressing gender-specific issues might also involve talking to a doctor about whether specific treatments or medications can help balance hormones or manage sleep disorders effectively.

Mental health plays an important role in sleep quality for both men and women. Stress, anxiety, and depression can rob anyone of good sleep. Recognizing the signs of these conditions and seeking the right treatment can improve sleep and overall well-being.

Understanding these differences isn't just about pinpointing problems—it's about creating solutions tailored to individual needs. Whether it's considering the impact of hormones, the likelihood of certain sleep disorders, or the specific challenges that come with each stage of life, recognizing and addressing these nuances can lead to better sleep and, by extension, better health.

9.3 Coping with Irregular Work Hours

If you work irregular hours, this can be another significant factor affecting the quality of your sleep. Whether you're working night shifts, rotating schedules, or irregular hours, finding the opportunity to get quality sleep can be a real challenge. These unconventional hours often conflict with your body's natural circadian rhythm, which is designed to tell you when to sleep and when to be awake.

Despite these challenges, there are still effective strategies to help you make the most of your workday and achieve better sleep. Creating a consistent routine is one of the first steps to managing sleep with irregular work hours. While consistency and irregular hours may seem incompatible, there is a way to manage them effectively without compromising your health.

Strive to maintain a consistent sleep schedule on both workdays and weekends. For example, if you wake up at 7 a.m. on Friday, aim to do the same on Saturday. This helps train your body to initiate a natural sleep response at specific times of the day, making it easier to fall asleep even when your schedule seems out of sync.

Next, create an optimal sleep environment. Invest in blackout curtains or a quality sleep mask, especially if you need to sleep during daylight hours. Keep the room quiet and peaceful—earplugs can be invaluable if you live in a noisy area. The goal is to signal to your body that it's time to rest, regardless of what's happening outside.

Now, let's talk about naps. Strategic napping can benefit shift workers by boosting alertness without throwing off your primary sleep cycle. Before starting your shift, take a short nap (around 20-30 minutes), but just be sure not to nap too close to your next sleep period as it might make it harder to fall asleep later.

Then, there's managing diet and exercise to avoid sleep disruptions. As much as possible, always avoid hearty or heavy meals and caffeine when it's late in the evening. You can also try to get some physical activity in, but like with eating, don't do it too close to when you plan to sleep. Exercise wakes your body up and can make it harder to wind down if done right before bed.

Finally, it's essential to communicate with your family or housemates about your schedule. They can support you by helping you maintain a quiet environment and understanding your sleep needs. Communicating your needs to the people around you and knowing that your home is conducive to rest can ease the stress of trying to sleep at odd hours. Managing sleep with irregular hours can be challenging, and finding what works best for you might require some experimentation.

However, with thoughtful planning and a few adjustments, you can establish a routine that provides the restorative sleep your body and mind need.

9.4 Sleep Strategies for Travelers

If you often travel across different time zones, you've likely faced your share of sleep challenges. Jet lag, unfamiliar environments, and the overall stress of travel can disrupt your sleep routine. But with the right strategies, you can still get quality rest while on the road.

Let's first talk about jet lag, which is your body's clock being out of sync with the local time. An intelligent way to minimize this disorientation is to adjust your schedule before leaving. If you're heading east, start going to bed and waking up a little earlier each day for a few days before your trip. If you're westward-bound, do the opposite. This pre-adjustment can lessen the shock to your system once you arrive.

Once you're on the plane, especially a long one, getting into a movie marathon might sound tempting, but consider settling down in your seat and resting first. An eye mask, a pair of earplugs, or even noise-canceling headphones can be absolute lifesavers. If it's nighttime at your current destination, try to sleep by making use of what you've learned so far. If it's daytime, do your best to stay awake. Mimicking the routine of your destination can help you adjust faster once you land.

Next, when you check into your hotel, set up an environment that's fit for sleep. This means adjusting the room's temperature to be a bit cooler (or warmer if it's too cold), closing the curtains to block out light, and ensuring it's as quiet as possible. If the hotel is noisy, ask for a room change—higher floors tend to be more peaceful. Bring a familiar item from home with you, like a favorite pillow or blanket, which can make an unfamiliar bed more comforting. Also, adjust your meals and drinks to match your destination's local time.

Even while traveling, there's always time for a bit of exercise. It doesn't have to be strenuous—a casual walk to explore the area or a quick workout at the hotel gym can be enough to help you wind down. Additionally, getting some natural daylight can help reset your internal clock and keep your sleep schedule on track.

Finally, always strive to maintain a routine. Even in a different place, keeping to your usual bedtime rituals helps you wind down. Sticking to your usual bedtime routine, even when you're far from home, can help you relax and transition smoothly into sleep. Carefully preparing for these trips and adapting to any situation appropriately will allow you to make the most out of your sleep and wake cycles.

Chapter 10

The Science of Dreams

Dreaming is an activity that has fascinated and mystified researchers and scientists for centuries. Depending on the cultural practices and beliefs, the interpretation of dreams, in general, ranged from believing that dreams were divine messages or *prophecies* to how dreams are a reflection of our unconscious mind.

It wasn't until the 1960s—after REM sleep was first discovered in the 1950s and then further researched—that a new theory on the strong association between dreams and memory consolidation was opened: how our nightly escapades are an important way of processing and storing information. This chapter will focus more on how dreams affect your sleep and waking life, as well as provide solutions for resolving issues that come with dreaming.

10.1 Dreams and Memory Consolidation

While our bodies rest, our brains sort through the day's experiences, focusing on what's essential. This process is particularly active during the REM sleep stage, characterized by heightened brain activity and vivid dreaming.

During REM sleep, the brain's hippocampus, responsible for forming new memories, collaborates with the neocortex, where long-term memories are stored. This interaction ensures that the day's learnings are stabilized and integrated into our overall knowledge framework. However, individuals who are deprived of REM sleep will exhibit impaired memory retention and cognitive function—students who get ample REM sleep after studying tend to perform better in exams than those who lack this critical sleep phase—emphasizing the need for a balanced sleep cycle to optimize learning and memory retention.

Dreams play a pivotal role in emotional processing; these allow the brain to work through complex feelings and help us manage stress and anxiety. This means that having nightmares, which are often linked to unresolved emotional conflicts, can provide insights into our subconscious struggles. By addressing these issues within the dreaming state, the brain can better prepare us to cope with them in our waking lives.

10.2 Common Forms of Dreams

Dreams can come in several forms. One of them is the recurring dreams, which repeat themselves over time, often with similar themes or narratives. These dreams can indicate unresolved issues or persistent concerns in the dreamer's life. They serve as a signal from the subconscious that there is something needing attention.

In terms of psychology, recurring dreams can be understood as the brain's way of processing ongoing problems or emotions, like how a dream about being unprepared for an exam might reflect real-life anxieties about competence and performance. Paying close attention to the content and frequency of these dreams will allow you to gain valuable insights into your emotional and psychological state, thus reducing the recurrence of these dreams.

Other than recurring dreams, there are universal dreams, which are common dreams that appear across different cultures and personal backgrounds. These themes often carry significant meanings related to our subconscious minds. Here are some examples:

- **Falling**: Dreams about falling can be associated with feelings of insecurity, instability, or fear of failure. They can indicate that the dreamer is experiencing a loss of control in some area of their life.

- **Flying**: Flying dreams are often seen as positive, symbolizing freedom, escape, or a desire to rise above challenges. They reflect a sense of empowerment and the ability to overcome obstacles.

- **Being Chased**: This theme typically signifies avoidance or fear. Dreams of being chased suggest that the dreamer is trying to evade a situation or emotion that they find threatening or stressful.

Interpreting these common themes can provide a deeper understanding of the dreamer's inner world or subconscious mind. Analyzing these types of dreams and their meanings will allow you to better perceive your subconscious and address the underlying emotions that influence your daily life.

10.3 Restorative Lucid Dreaming

Lucid dreaming, where the dreamer is aware they are dreaming and can often control the dream narrative, is a fascinating phenomenon that can significantly impact sleep quality and mental well-being.

Lucid dreaming occurs when the dreamer becomes conscious of their dream state and can influence the course of their dreams. This awareness typically arises during the REM stage of sleep, where brain activity is high, resembling wakefulness—it allows for an extraordinary experience where the dreamer can explore their subconscious mind, confront fears, and maybe even practice real-life skills in a safe dream environment.

This unique form of dreaming has intrigued scientists and psychologists for decades, leading to extensive research on its mechanisms and benefits.

Techniques to Encourage Restorative Dreaming

Achieving lucid dreams can enhance sleep quality by providing a sense of control and reducing the frequency of nightmares.

There are several ways to allow yourself to experience restorative lucid dreaming, many of which would require a bit of preparation, so here are some techniques to prepare yourself for restorative dreaming:

- **Reality Checks**: Perform regular reality checks throughout the day, such as looking at your hands or checking the time, to build the habit of questioning your reality. This habit often carries over into dreams, increasing the likelihood of becoming lucid.

- **Mnemonic Induction of Lucid Dreams (MILD)**: Repeat the phrase "I will know I am dreaming" or something similar to reinforce the intention of becoming lucid. Visualization of becoming lucid in a recent dream can also be effective.

- **Wake Back to Bed (WBTB)**: Set an alarm to wake up after 4-6 hours of sleep, stay awake for a short period, and then go back to sleep. This method increases the chances of entering REM sleep while maintaining some level of consciousness.

Properly preparing yourself for lucid dreaming means that you're encouraging your mind to be more comfortable knowing that you're dreaming, which significantly lessens the chances of a nightmare from occurring and allows your body to relax better.

Dream Journaling for Lucid Dreaming

Dream journaling is a practice where you record your dreams after waking up to capture the details while one is still fresh. This habit not only aids in recalling dreams more vividly but also provides valuable insights into the subconscious mind.

Regularly writing down dreams significantly enhances dream recall—noting the details of dreams can allow you to remember them over time better and, eventually, remember even finer details when you're awake.

This practice also serves as a gateway to the subconscious, helping to uncover hidden thoughts and emotions. Over time, patterns and recurring themes may emerge, offering deeper understanding and self-awareness.

Dream journaling is particularly beneficial for those interested in lucid dreaming: keeping a consistent record of dreams increases awareness of dream patterns, making it easier to achieve lucidity in future dreams.

It may also allow you to have a deeper look into your own subconscious and psyche, which could possibly provide you with an emotional or spiritual look and clarity of the events and situations that you're currently experiencing in your waking life.

Here are some steps you can follow to start with your dream journal:

1. Keep within arm's reach of your bed so you can write immediately upon waking.

2. Jot down everything you remember, even if it's just fragments. You can include as many details as possible, such as colors, emotions, people, places, and any symbols or strange occurrences.

Periodically review your entries to identify patterns or recurring themes. Do this consistently—make it a habit, even if some mornings you only remember a small snippet.

Lucid Dreaming in Recent Studies

Research has explored the mechanisms and benefits of lucid dreaming, with studies suggesting that lucid dreaming involves heightened activity in the prefrontal cortex, the brain region associated with self-awareness and decision-making.

This increase in brain activity is what differentiates lucid dreaming from regular dreaming and allows for conscious control. The advantages of lucid dreaming extend beyond the dream state—lucid dreamers often report improved problem-solving skills, enhanced creativity, and reduced anxiety.

By confronting and managing fears within dreams, individuals can lessen the frequency and intensity of nightmares to have better sleep and overall mental health.

Lucid dreaming, in this regard, can be a potential tool for improving sleep quality and emotional well-being by having control of your subconscious mind to better your waking life.

10.4 Parasomnia

Dreams aren't always peaceful, however. While dreams can provide an insightful look into our subconscious and even offer therapeutic benefits, parasomnias represent the darker side of our sleep experiences.

These sleep disorders involve unusual and often disruptive physical events or behaviors that occur during sleep, all of which could significantly affect the quality of rest and overall well-being.

Parasomnias are sleep disorders that heavily involve unusual behaviors, movements, emotions, and perceptions, as well as dreams that occur during the different sleep stages.

These are more than just bad dreams or occasional sleepwalking; they include a wide range of behaviors that can impact a person's safety, mental health, and quality of sleep because of how intense they *can* become.

People with parasomnias may act out their dreams, engage in activities they don't remember, or experience vivid sensations that disrupt their sleep. These disorders are puzzling, even to those who experience them.

Often, people with parasomnias have no memory of their actions or behaviors, leaving them confused, terrified, or embarrassed when they wake up.

10.5 Types of Parasomnias

There are several common types of parasomnias, each with unique characteristics and challenges:

Sleepwalking (Somnambulism) and RBD

Sleepwalking is perhaps the most well-known parasomnia. It involves getting up and walking around while still in a deep stage of sleep. Sleepwalkers may perform complex behaviors, like going outside or rearranging furniture, without any awareness.

Since sleepwalking occurs during deep sleep, waking someone during an episode can be challenging, and they usually have no recollection of the event.

On the other hand, RBD or REM Sleep Behavior Disorder is when a person physically acts out their dreams, often in violent or intense ways. As the name suggests, it happens during REM sleep—when most dreaming happens.

RBD can cause a person to kick, punch, or shout. It can be dangerous, as the person may unknowingly harm themselves or a sleep partner.

Both sleepwalking and RBD can become dangerous if these disorders aren't properly acknowledged.

To prevent possible injuries and other bodily risks, here are some safety and management tips that could keep you or the concerned individual safe:

- Ensure a safe sleeping environment by removing sharp objects as well as padding the edges of nightstands, headboards, and other furniture.
- Secure the bedroom by locking doors and windows.
- If possible, place the mattress on the floor or use a bed rail to prevent falls.
- Set up alarms or bells on bedroom doors to alert others if the person gets up during the night.

Taking these steps to prevent injuries will help you, or the person with this parasomnia, sleep better at night.

However, in some cases, medication may be prescribed to manage more severe sleepwalking and RBD episodes.

Sleep Talking (Somniloquy)

Sleep talking is a milder form of parasomnia where a person talks, laughs, or even has full conversations while asleep. It can range from simple sounds to full sentences. While it's generally harmless, it can be disruptive for sleep partners and is often associated with other sleep disorders or periods of stress.

Confusional Arousals

This form of parasomnia involves disorientation, confusion, and sometimes inappropriate behavior upon waking. A person may appear awake but act confused or startled. These episodes are often brief and occur during deep sleep stages, leaving the person unaware of their behavior.

Night Terrors and Sleep Paralysis

Unlike nightmares, sleep terrors, or night terrors, typically occur in the first half of the night, during deep sleep. A person who experiences night terrors may suddenly sit up, scream, thrash around, or appear terrified. They often have no memory of the episode upon waking.

Meanwhile, Sleep paralysis occurs when a person becomes temporarily unable to move or speak as they fall asleep or are in the process of waking up. During these episodes, many people feel a sense of fear or the sensation of pressure on their chest. Although these parasomnias are not essentially harmful, both sleep disorders can be frightening to experience and are often associated with stress or irregular sleep schedules.

However, the difference between these two sleep disorders is that night terrors are more common in children, while sleep paralysis is often seen occurring in adolescents and adults.

Nightmares

Our brain uses dreams to process both positive and negative information, as well as cope with daily stressors and other major life changes—including unresolved conflicts, intense emotions, and traumatic events.

Once you're exposed to negative experiences, the information and experiences gathered in your waking hours will be interpreted by your brain as nightmares, a type of dream that is an unpleasant emotional regulation.

However, unlike night terrors and sleep paralysis, nightmares are easier to manage and are almost predictable depending on the circumstances.

Below are tips and strategies you can take to manage nightmares:

- **Realize it's a dream**: If you can recognize that you are in a nightmare, remind yourself that it's not real and that you are safe. This awareness can sometimes help reduce the fear.

- **Focus on breathing**: Calm your mind by taking slow, deep breaths. This can help reduce the intensity of the nightmare and may even help you wake up.

- **Change the dream**: If you're aware that you're dreaming, try to change the narrative of the nightmare. Visualize a positive or safe outcome, or focus on a different scene entirely.

- **Ground yourself**: If you wake up from a nightmare, use grounding techniques to bring yourself back to reality. This can include focusing on your surroundings, touching a familiar object, or repeating a calming mantra.

Depending on whether you've experienced nightmares before or not, these tips may sound hard or even silly at first. But as someone who has experienced nightmares due to work stress and other encounters in real life, learning how to manage my dreams and nightmares has been one of the best seemingly unnecessary, necessary lifehacks I have ever had the fortune to even know about.

Developing an understanding of an unpredictable aspect of our sleep, such as dreams and the like, can heavily impact the way we approach our nightly routines.

Chapter 11

Innovations in
Sleep Science

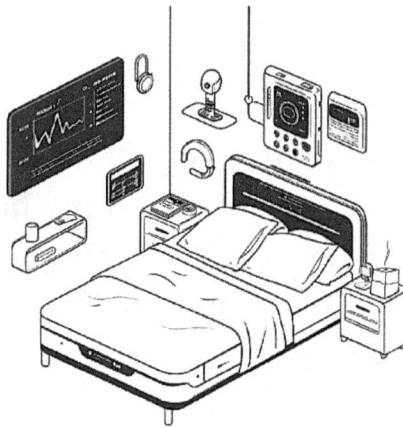

In this chapter, we'll explore the latest research and innovations in sleep science—examining potential causes of sleep disorders and how advancements in technology and medicine can help us improve sleep patterns for better rest.

11.1 Latest Research on Sleep and Health

Recent studies by doctors and scientists have significantly advanced our understanding of the relationship between cognitive functions and different stages of sleep. While the widely recommended sleep duration for adults is seven to nine hours, emerging research suggests that the quality of sleep—particularly the time spent in light, deep, and REM sleep cycles—is more crucial than the total hours slept.

During our nightly sleep cycles, the brain filters out waste and organizes memories while efficiently focusing on repair, leading to better moods and overall well-being. However, when sleep quality is poor, even minor problems upon waking can feel overwhelming and difficult to manage. Our health can be heavily affected by the quality of our sleep.

There has also been growing evidence that consistently having poor sleep quality can result in a higher probability of long-lasting diseases like cardiovascular disease, obesity, and diabetes. Better sleep can help regulate hormones that control appetite, metabolism, and glucose processing. It also plays an important role in maintaining a healthy immune system—in short, poor sleep means our health becomes more compromised and vulnerable to illnesses.

Sleep, in relation to Alzheimer's, is another area of research that demonstrates the potential for sleep to combat neurodegenerative disease. The way our brains remove waste from the system, known as the glymphatic system, is primarily active during sleep—which might help prevent the buildup of amyloid plaques linked to Alzheimer's.

11.2 Personalized Medicine and Genomics

Personalized medical treatments for sleep disorders were developed after researchers studied genetic markers that influence sleep patterns, allowing them to create tailored approaches for each individual. This means that for every unique sleep challenge a patient faces, there can now be an equally customized solution specifically designed for them.

Everyone has their own unique traits—particularly when it comes to sleep. While most people struggle without eight hours of sleep, some can thrive on just a few hours. This means that our genetic makeup directly affects our sleep patterns; with that, the importance of understanding genomics and personalized medicine has begun to radically change how doctors and sleep specialists provide individualized treatment to those with sleeping disorders.

The study of our genomes—called genomics—uncovers the genetic variations that explain why we sleep the way we do. Essentially, the variations in each person's genes can make some people do better in the morning while others can stay awake throughout the night. An examination of our genetic code can explain our current sleep habits, which could lead sleep specialists and doctors to build customized sleep recommendations. Once your genetic information is completely analyzed, you can live a life more tailored to your daily schedule, diet, and environment to sync perfectly with your natural sleep-wake cycle.

As long as you follow the holistic sleep plans and routines that consider everything from your genetic predispositions to your current health status, age, and stress levels. This approach could transform the treatment of sleep disorders.

11.3 The Future of Sleep Technology

As we move into an era where technology can actively fine-tune the quality of a person's sleep, it's not surprising to think that there will be a time when "perfect" sleep could become increasingly easy to achieve for people.

Imagine slipping into bed at night, and your mattress adjusts its firmness based on your body's pressure points—maybe the temperature is also constantly changing to keep you snug yet cool enough for perfect sleep. This isn't a distant dream; it's the direction sleep tech is headed, and companies are developing intelligent beds that can do all this and more, from gently waking you up at the best part of your sleep cycle with soft vibrations and-or warmth rather than a jarring alarm clock buzz.

And think about wearables—they're getting smarter, too. Future devices could predict sleep disturbances before they happen by monitoring signs like the variability in heart rate and subtle changes in your waking breathing patterns. If those wearable smart devices are connected to your room, they could automatically make adjustments like dimming the lights or activating soundscapes that promote deeper sleep, all tailored just for you. Something that's one step ahead, making sure you get the best rest possible.

However, in terms of being a step further, there are some apps and programs that can track sleep and use AI to analyze patterns, providing personalized advice on how to tweak your habits for better sleep. Some apps can connect with other pro-sleep devices and wearables in your home to create the comfiest, perfect sleep environment.

Additionally, something that is, and has been, even several steps further since 1838 is the promising field of augmented and virtual reality. It's taken nearly two centuries for technology like these to develop to where it is now: from the invention of the stereoscope to the most mind-bending engineered advancements of today that could transform the pre-sleep routine by immersing you in calming environments. A person can easily detach from day-to-day stresses using a VR headset and then be transported to a serene beach or a quiet forest to wind down. All of this has the possibility of making it easier to fall asleep.

As for neurotechnology—there's a good chance it could possibly enhance brain function as you sleep, improving memory consolidation or learning processes. This means you could potentially *learn* new information or stabilize learned information while you snooze, essentially leveraging how sleep affects the mind to the nth degree.

Sleep technology is becoming more integrated and holistic. The ecosystem of devices that support all aspects of your sleep could mean significant improvements in public health, given the crucial role sleep plays in overall well-being.

All these advancements promise to not only make good sleep more accessible but also transform how we think about and experience our nightly recharge.

Chapter 12

Professional and Medical Sleep Solutions

Sometimes, even with our best attempts at lifestyle changes and home remedies, sleep can still be elusive, which can be admittingly frustrating for most people.

When this happens, it may be time to explore professional and medical solutions. There is absolutely no shame in seeking help from experts. Understanding when to seek help from sleep experts, the types of specialists available, and the treatments they can offer.

The final chapter of this book will detail essential steps towards achieving restorative sleep with the help of medical professionals, from navigating the options for sleep medications to understanding what a visit to a sleep clinic entails.

12.1 Seeking Medical Help

Poor sleep has the potential to heavily affect everything from your overall mood and energy to your mental clarity and capacity to manage stress.

So, if sleeping poorly is becoming your norm, it's essential to take it seriously.

Another red flag is if you feel excessively sleepy during the day, even after what you thought was a whole night's sleep. This could indicate sleep apnea or another sleep disorder preventing you from getting deep, restorative sleep.

Symptoms like loud snoring, waking up gasping for air, or feeling like choking in your sleep are cues to see a professional.

Also, if you notice that your struggle with sleep is starting to impact your daily life—like causing you to feel irritable, depressed, or anxious—it's time to talk to someone. Sleep problems can be the cause and symptom of mental health issues, and addressing one can help improve the other.

Chronic pain that keeps you awake is another serious reason to seek help. Pain management and sleep improvement often go hand-in-hand, and a healthcare provider can help you tackle both.

Visiting your primary care doctor can help rule out any underlying conditions that might mess with your sleep, or they might refer you to a sleep specialist.

Sleep specialists are experts when it comes to diagnosing and treating sleep disorders, using tools like sleep studies to get a clear picture of what's happening while you sleep.

12.2 Sleep Health Medical Specialists

Here's a list of the various sleep specialists that you could book an appointment to:

Primary Care Physician (PCP): They're often the first stop for any health concern, including sleep issues. Your PCP can check for general health problems affecting your sleep, like thyroid issues or diabetes. They can also offer initial advice on sleep hygiene and, if needed, direct you to more specialized help, like a sleep specialist.

Sleep Specialist: These doctors have specific training in sleep medicine, which means they're experts at dealing with sleep disorders like insomnia, sleep apnea, restless legs syndrome, and more. They work in sleep clinics where they can conduct studies to monitor your sleep patterns in detail, usually through an overnight stay. Afterward, they tailor treatments specifically for you depending on how well you slept the night before.

Neurologist: If your sleep issues are related to neurological conditions like narcolepsy or epilepsy, neurologists can analyze your brain and nervous system to check for any sleep disturbances.

Pulmonologist: For those who have breathing issues, such as sleep apnea, these doctors are specialists in lung and respiratory health. They can provide treatments like continuous positive airway pressure (CPAP), which are machines that help keep your airway open while you sleep, preventing the dangerous pauses in breathing that characterize sleep apnea.

Psychiatrist / Psychologist: These are doctors who specialize in sleep disorders relating to mental disorders like anxiety and depression. These specialized doctors can offer therapies like CBT-I, which has already been proven to be highly effective.

Dentist: This might sound a bit out of left field, but dentists can help with sleep by providing devices for sleep apnea or snoring. These devices adjust the position of your mouth or jaw during sleep to keep your airway open and are often an alternative for those who can't tolerate CPAP machines. They can also inspect your mouth to see if toothaches or other oral issues may have been the cause of your sleep problems.

As you can see, a whole array of specialists is ready to help you get a better night's sleep, each offering different expertise that could help find and resolve the root cause of your sleep issues.

12.3 Preparing for a Sleep Clinic Visit

A sleep clinic is where experts dig deep into your sleep issues. Often, overnight stays are required, during which they monitor everything from your brain waves to your heart rate while you snooze.

Gathering a bit of info beforehand can really help both you and your doctors prepare for an in-depth examination.

Start with a sleep diary. A couple of weeks before your appointment, jot down your sleep habits—list down the times you sleep and wake up, how often you wake during the night, and how you feel in the morning. This kind of info can give the specialists a clearer picture of what might be going wrong.

Next, consider your health history. The doctors will want to know not just about your sleep but also about any conditions you have or medications you take that could be affecting it. Bring a list of your medications, including any over-the-counter ones, since something as simple as an allergy pill could be contributing to your sleep issues.

Then, there's the questionnaire you'll likely need to fill out when you arrive at the clinic. It might cover enough ground—everything from your lifestyle to your nightly routines. Answering this questionnaire honestly and thoroughly in your responses can provide crucial clues in diagnosing and treating your sleep issues.

If you're recommended to stay overnight, pack as if you were staying at a hotel for a night. Bring comfortable pajamas, your toothbrush, and maybe even your favorite pillow if that helps you sleep better. Clinics usually try to make the environment as comfortable as possible, resembling a typical bedroom, to ensure your sleep study is as close to your real sleeping experience. It's also a good idea to avoid caffeine and alcohol on the day of your sleep study. Both can significantly alter your sleep patterns. Also, try to keep your daytime routine as normal as possible so the survey accurately reflects your typical night's sleep.

Once you're at the clinic, don't be shy about asking questions—knowing what kinds of tests will be run, how the equipment works, and when you'll get the results can ease your mind. The more you understand the process, the more comfortable you'll be.

Finally, remember that the goal of the visit is to help you sleep better. This might be just the first step in addressing your sleep issues, so it's important to keep an open line of communication with the sleep specialists and follow up with them about the results and next steps.

Conclusion

You've finally reached the end of the book, and we've touched on a variety of different approaches—from diet, routine, environment, and how all of that affects sleep. This journey towards better sleep wasn't just about occasional adjustments and committing to long-term changes that enhance your life's quality.

Let's do a quick recap on the essential strategies and tips that can transform your nightly rest.

Throughout this book, we've established consistent healthy routines and sleep hygiene and even laid out the impact of diet and exercise on sleep quality. We've also looked at the role of technology in monitoring and improving our sleep patterns and the importance of creating a sleep-conducive environment. Each strategy is a piece of the puzzle, helping to construct a complete picture of what good sleep looks like.

Acknowledging how getting proper sleep impacts our life overall—from our health to mood—is all part of making sure we're feeling fully rested. Sleep must be prioritized, **not** sacrificed for more work or screen time. A good few hours of awake time might be nice and tempting, but sleep is a necessity that we should never take for granted. The benefits of sleep can and will influence every bit of our lives, including our relationships, productivity, and even the ability to remember things properly.

I encourage you to not just read about these changes—but to start implementing them as soon as you can. In fact, the best time you can implement these changes is tonight while the information is still fresh. However, it's always best to do this comfortably. Whether you adjust your evening routine, invest in blackout curtains, or set a stricter schedule, every small step is a leap toward better health. You don't have to overhaul your life overnight, of course. Even small, incremental changes can have profound effects over time as long as you can remain as consistent as you can while doing so at your own pace.

To conclude...

...Remember that attaining better sleep isn't just a mere possibility that's "just out of reach"—it **is** within your reach. Embrace the practices you've learned, but be patient with yourself. Let your journey towards better sleep strengthen every day.

Tonight could be your first step to a lifestyle of restful, peaceful sleep.

- Kiley Manning

Pass On the Gift of Restful Sleep

Now that you have the tools to conquer insomnia, boost your energy, and optimize your health, it's time to pass on what you've learned. Share your experience to help others find the same restful nights you now enjoy.

By leaving your honest review on Amazon, you can guide others struggling with sleep issues toward the answers they need. Your review could be the key that unlocks better sleep and brighter days for someone else.

Thank you for being part of this journey. When we share our knowledge, we help others find the rest they deserve—and you're playing a vital role in that.

- *Kiley Manning*

References

Akerstedt, T., & Wright, K. P. (2009). Sleep loss and fatigue in shift work and shift work disorder. Sleep Medicine Clinics, 4(2), 257-271. https://doi.org/10.1016/j.jsmc.2009.03.001

Ancoli-Israel, S., & Roth, T. (1999). Characteristics of insomnia in the United States: Results of the 1991 National Sleep Foundation Survey. Sleep, 22(Suppl 2), S347-S353. https://doi.org/10.1093/sleep/22.suppl_2.S347

Benca, R. M., Obermeyer, W. H., Thisted, R. A., & Gillin, J. C. (1992). Sleep and psychiatric disorders: A meta-analysis. Archives of General Psychiatry, 49(8), 651-668. https://doi.org/10.1001/archpsyc.1992.01820080059010

Bonnet, M. H., & Arand, D. L. (2010). Hyperarousal and insomnia: State of the science. Sleep Medicine Reviews, 14(1), 9-15. https://doi.org/10.1016/j.smrv.2009.05.002

Cappuccio, F. P., D'Elia, L., Strazzullo, P., & Miller, M. A. (2010). Sleep duration and all-cause mortality: A systematic review and meta-analysis of prospective studies. Sleep, 33(5), 585-592. https://doi.org/10.1093/sleep/33.5.585

Carskadon, M. A., & Dement, W. C. (2011). Normal human sleep: An overview. In M. H. Kryger, T. Roth, & W. C. Dement (Eds.), Principles and practice of sleep medicine (5th ed., pp. 16-26). Elsevier.

Chokroverty, S. (2017). Sleep disorders medicine: Basic science, technical considerations, and clinical aspects (4th ed.). Springer.

Czeisler, C. A. (2015). Perspective: Casting light on sleep deficiency. Nature, 527, S8-S9. https://doi.org/10.1038/527S8a

Dinges, D. F., Pack, F., Williams, K., Gillen, K. A., Powell, J. W., Ott, G. E., ... & Pack, A. I. (1997). Cumulative sleepiness, mood disturbance, and psychomotor vigilance performance decrements during a week of sleep restricted to 4-5 hours per night. Sleep, 20(4), 267-277. https://doi.org/10.1093/sleep/20.4.267

Foster, R. G., & Kreitzman, L. (2017). Circadian rhythms: A very short introduction. Oxford University Press.

Harvey, A. G., Murray, G., Chandler, R. A., & Soehner, A. M. (2011). Sleep disturbance as transdiagnostic: Consideration of neurobiological mechanisms. Clinical Psychology Review, 31(2), 225-235. https://doi.org/10.1016/j.cpr.2010.04.003

Hirshkowitz, M., Whiton, K., Albert, S. M., Alessi, C., Bruni, O., DonCarlos, L., & Adams Hillard, P. J. (2015). National Sleep Foundation's sleep time duration recommendations: Methodology and results summary. Sleep Health, 1(1), 40-43. https://doi.org/10.1016/j.sleh.2014.12.010 https://doi.org/10.1097/01.JPN.0000319095.40960.23

Irwin, M. R. (2015). Why sleep is important for health: A psychoneuroimmunology perspective. Annual Review of Psychology, 66(1), 143-172. https://doi.org/10.1146/annurev-psych-010213-115205

Kripke, D. F., Langer, R. D., & Kline, L. E. (2012). Hypnotics' association with mortality or cancer: A matched cohort study. BMJ Open, 2(1), e000850. https://doi.org/10.1136/bmjopen-2012-000850

Morin, C. M., & Benca, R. (2012). Chronic insomnia. The Lancet, 379(9821), 1129-1141. https://doi.org/10.1016/S0140-6736(11)60750-2

Owens, J. (2008). Sleep loss and fatigue in healthcare professionals. The Journal of Perinatal & Neonatal Nursing, 22(2), 92-100.

Perlis, M. L., & Gehrman, P. (2013). Insomnia and its treatment. Sleep Medicine Clinics, 8(2), 229-240. https://doi.org/10.1016/j.jsmc.2013.04.009

Rasch, B., & Born, J. (2013). About sleep's role in memory. Physiological Reviews, 93(2), 681-766. https://doi.org/10.1152/physrev.00032.2012

Riemann, D., & Spiegelhalder, K. (2009). The neurobiology of insomnia: An update. Nature Reviews Neurology, 5(5), 216-225. https://doi.org/10.1038/nrneurol.2009.23

Riemann, D., Nissen, C., Palagini, L., Otte, A., Perlis, M. L., & Spiegelhalder, K. (2015). The neurobiology, investigation, and treatment of chronic insomnia. The Lancet Neurology, 14(5), 547-558. https://doi.org/10.1016/S1474-4422(15)00021-6

Sateia, M. J. (2014). International classification of sleep disorders-third edition: Highlights and modifications. Chest, 146(5), 1387-1394. https://doi.org/10.1378/chest.14-0970

Schwartz, J. R., & Roth, T. (2008). Neurophysiology of sleep and wakefulness: Basic science and clinical implications. Current Neuropharmacology, 6(4), 367-378. https://doi.org/10.2174/157015908787386050

Shapiro, C. M., & Dement, W. C. (1993). ABC of sleep disorders. BMJ Publishing Group.

Siegel, J. M. (2005). Clues to the functions of mammalian sleep. Nature, 437(7063), 1264-1271. https://doi.org/10.1038/nature04285

Spiegel, K., Tasali, E., Penev, P., & Van Cauter, E. (2004). Brief communication: Sleep curtailment in healthy young men is associated with decreased leptin levels, elevated ghrelin levels, and increased hunger and appetite. Annals of Internal Medicine, 141(11), 846-850. https://doi.org/10.7326/0003-4819-141-11-200412070-00008

Van Cauter, E., Leproult, R., & Plat, L. (2000). Age-related changes in slow wave sleep and REM sleep and relationship with growth hormone and cortisol levels in healthy men. Journal of the American Medical Association, 284(7), 861-868. https://doi.org/10.1001/jama.284.7.861

Van Dongen, H. P., Maislin, G., Mullington, J. M., & Dinges, D. F. (2003). The cumulative cost of additional wakefulness: Dose-response effects on neurobehavioral functions and sleep physiology from chronic sleep restriction and total sleep deprivation. Sleep, 26(2), 117-126. https://doi.org/10.1093/sleep/26.2.117

Walker, M. (2017). Why we sleep: Unlocking the power of sleep and dreams. Scribner.

Wichniak, A., Wierzbicka, A., & Jernajczyk, W. (2013). Sleep and antidepressant treatment. Current Pharmaceutical Design, 19(14), 2428-2449. https://doi.org/10.2174/1381612811319140003

Zhdanova, I. V., Wurtman, R. J., Lynch, H. J., Ives, J. R., Dollins, A. B., Morabito, C., ... & Schomer, D. L. (1995). Sleep-inducing effects of low doses of melatonin ingested in the evening. Clinical Pharmacology & Therapeutics, 57(5), 552-558. https://doi.org/10.1016/0009-9236(95)90291-0

www.ingramcontent.com/pod-product-compliance
Lightning Source LLC
Chambersburg PA
CBHW070112030426
42335CB00016B/2121